THE **GOOD** VICES

The

GOOD
VICES

From Beer to Sex, the Surprising Truth About What's Actually Good for You

DR. HARRY OFGANG
AND ERIK OFGANG

A TARCHERPERIGEE BOOK

tarcherperigee

An imprint of Penguin Random House LLC
penguinrandomhouse.com

TarcherPerigee with tp colophon is a registered trademark of
Penguin Random House LLC.

Most TarcherPerigee books are available at special quantity discounts for bulk
purchase for sales promotions, premiums, fund-raising, and educational needs.
Special books or book excerpts also can be created to fit specific needs.
For details, write: SpecialMarkets@penguinrandomhouse.com.

Library of Congress Cataloging-in-Publication Data

Names: Ofgang, Harry, author. | Ofgang, Erik, author.
Title: The good vices: from beer to sex, the surprising truth about what's
actually good for you / Dr. Harry Ofgang and Erik Ofgang.
Description: New York: TarcherPerigee, 2019. | Includes bibliographical references.
Identifiers: LCCN 2018057940| ISBN 9780143131960 (paperback) |
ISBN 9780525503750 (ebook)
Subjects: LCSH: Nutrition—Popular works. | Health—Popular works. |
Diet—Popular works. | BISAC: HEALTH & FITNESS / Healthy Living. |
HEALTH & FITNESS / Naturopathy. | HEALTH & FITNESS / Nutrition.
Classification: LCC RA784 .O34 2019 | DDC 613.2—dc23
LC record available at https://lccn.loc.gov/2018057940

Printed in the United States of America
1   3   5   7   9   10   8   6   4   2

Book design by Kristin del Rosario

To my mom and dad, Ethel and Nathan "Nussie,"
who were with me every day,
even when I lived across the Atlantic three thousand miles away.

To my grandparents, who gave me not only my parents
but the warmest, most loving childhood, and who shared
the joys of good vices with me each and every day, literally,
as we grew up in their house in Brownsville, Brooklyn.

To my uncle Foxy and aunt Billy, who introduced me
to lots of good (and bad) vices.

To my brother Bob, who gave me my first car,
a V8 Mercury convertible; my first baseball mitt;
and my first dog, Buddy.

To my four children, two of whom I had the joy of delivering
at home, for showing me the promise of God in their eyes
the moment they were born.

To my and man's best friends, the Orsos and Hondos of the world.

And most of all to Patty, the ultimate "Good (and a little bad) Vice."
—DR. HARRY OFGANG

To Corinne and my family, without whom there would be
no vices good enough to enjoy.
—ERIK

Men are more easily governed through their vices than through their virtues.

—Napoléon

CONTENTS

Contents

THE **GOOD** VICES

INTRODUCTION

■ ■ ■

The art of medicine consists of amusing
the patient while nature cures the disease.
—VOLTAIRE

A doctor's role is simple. As Samuel Hahnemann, the pioneering German physician and founder of homeopathic medicine, explained more than two hundred years ago: "The physician's high and only purpose is to restore the sick to health, to cure, as it is termed."

Natural medicine works by metaphorically lighting a fuse, which helps ignite or supercharge the body's defense mechanism or vital force. Health is first, health is second, health is third. This includes mental, emotional, and physical health.

But what is health? As we learned many years ago on the beautiful Greek island of Alonissos in the Aegean Sea, from our friend, world-renowned author and teacher George Vithoulkas: *Health is freedom.*

Physical health is freedom from undue pain and other symptoms of disease. Emotional health is freedom to experience the full range of emotions from sadness to happiness, while not being trapped or stuck in any one emotion, negative or positive. For example, it is normal to feel grief and sadness after a breakup or the loss of a loved one, but it is not healthy to be trapped in negative emotions forever. Mental freedom includes freedom of thought, clarity of mind, and selfless creativity.

Finally, once we have physical, mental, and emotional health, we must have enough energy to enjoy our lives. And it's this last part, *enjoyment*, that includes some "good vices" and often gets left out of the healthy living equation.

The next time you're at the doctor's office, if she tells you to stop taking your medication and not to come back for a checkup so soon, you'd be confused. If she follows up by telling you that it's okay to eat some chocolate and fatty foods, enjoy a glass of beer or wine, or have lots of coffee, you'd think she was crazy, right? But in fact she would be doing something far too few medical professionals do: advising patients based on the latest available science.

Much of the health advice we receive today is misguided and based on old conventions rather than the latest research. To be healthy, we are led to believe that we must spend half our lives in doctors' offices, ingest a constant stream of narcotic-strength drugs, consume a Spartan diet, drink so-called health elixirs that look like witch's potions, and exercise with the intensity of an Olympic athlete and the joy of a KGB recruit. We must worry about the food we eat, the tests we don't take, and the pills we don't swallow. Above all, we must worry. And all that worry costs us dearly—monetarily, emotionally, and physically.

The goal of medicine should be to increase two things: the quality and the quantity of life. In other words, after seeing your doctor, are you going to live longer and have a better life? Conventional medicine often scares us by telling us what *might* happen if we don't use this or that drug, have this or that procedure, or take this or that test. Maybe they also should scare us by mentioning the potential risks associated with introducing these often unnecessary and unnatural substances and procedures into the body.

Our old friend and mentor, famed Argentinian physician, professor, and author Francisco Eizayaga, often said that "a good doctor never follows money, even though money may follow a good doctor." Yet the annual health-care expenditure in the United States is more than $3 trillion, or an average of close to $10,000 per person. Meanwhile, one study by researchers at Johns Hopkins Medicine estimated that more than 250,000 people die annually in the United States from medical mistakes or wrongdoing, making it the nation's third-leading cause of death behind only cancer and heart disease. If this estimate is correct, it means that going to the doctor or hospital and doing exactly as we're told may end up killing more of us each year than guns and automobile accidents. Let that sink in for a moment.[1] Starting in the mid-1990s, if you went to a doctor and complained of pain, you may have been given narcotic painkillers so strong, they were once reserved solely for in-hospital use for terminally ill patients. If you said it wasn't working and the pain was persisting, your dosage might have been increased. This pharmaceutical-industry-encouraged practice resulted in opioid use so aggressive that it has helped create a culture of addiction, claiming tens of thousands of lives a year. The prescription painkiller problem also has contributed to the nation's heroin epidemic, as estimates indicate that four out of every five heroin users started by misusing prescription opioids.

Opioid prescriptions may get the most press, but they are far from the only problem in medicine today. For example, currently more than a third of Americans take at least one prescription drug that has a side effect of depression, according to a study published in *JAMA*. Those who take such drugs—which include more than two hundred commonly prescribed medications—have higher rates of depression than those who don't. Many of these drugs also list suicidal symptoms as a side effect, and ironically some of them are supposed to treat depression.[2]

Yet the pharmaceutical industry remains a multibillion-dollar juggernaut with substantial influence over the U.S. Food and Drug Administration. Traditionally, a person who did not feel well would go to a physician, who would then try to figure out what was wrong and help restore the patient to a healthy state. Now we are told by one advertisement after another on prime-time TV to ask the doctor to give us a specific drug. We are by no means just throwing shade at conventional medicine, which of course can be indispensable and lifesaving. We are simply advocating greater objectivity and logic when it comes to the use of traditional medicine.

We also have some good news. Being healthy is easier, less worrisome, less expensive, and a whole lot more enjoyable than you think. In this book, we—Dr. Harry Ofgang, a prominent naturopathic physician with nearly forty years of experience, and his son Erik Ofgang, a food and health journalist—aim to boldly take readers where no health book has gone before, tearing down generations of myth and prejudice to provide an unflinching look at some of society's guilty pleasures that are not only okay but actually may help bolster our health.

While other health books focus on the "thou shalt nots," *The*

Good Vices is a "thou shalt" guide to healthy and happy living. Ancient Greek physician Hippocrates, the father of medicine, famously said, "Let food be thy medicine." Too often, contemporary medicine says to let worry and overprescribed drugs be thy medicine, but we say let good friends, family, food, nature, and happiness be thy medicine. And we suggest reminding your doctors of the words from the Hippocratic oath: "I will use those dietary regimens which will benefit my patients according to my greatest ability and judgment, and I will do no harm or injustice to them."

Throughout his nearly four-decade medical career, Dr. Ofgang has championed a more natural approach to health care. His grandfather, after whom he is named, was known as the neighborhood healer in turn-of-the-century Brooklyn. Though natural medicine is considered a "vice" by many conventional (allopathic) doctors, when used appropriately, in many cases it may be the better approach. Why not use a safe, gentle, natural method wherever possible and save the more toxic big guns (drugs and invasive procedures) for when they are really needed?

Over the course of his career, Dr. Ofgang studied common trends among his patients, particularly those who aged gracefully and in good health. He noticed many of his oldest and most active patients incorporated certain so-called vices into their daily routines. He found that regular moderate consumption of beer, wine, coffee, butter, cheese, pickles, fermented vegetables, and other delicious natural foods were often at the top of these patients' lists of daily rituals. He also noted that regularly enjoying these and other vices (and spices) while maintaining healthy and fun practices like walking outside, enjoying the company of friends and family, having hearty laughs, and listening to good music was often positively linked to a patient's overall health. In short, patients seemed to benefit from a host of nonprescription practices and certain so-called good vices that lead not only to happier lives but also to healthier ones.

Over the years, mainstream medical studies at respected institutions—from Harvard to Yale—have shown repeatedly that many of the foods and behaviors we've been warned to avoid all our lives may not really harm us, and when consumed or engaged in properly, actually may be beneficial. The list of good vices includes beverages like coffee, which research suggests can lower the risk of type 2 diabetes and possibly protect from Alzheimer's disease and dementia; foods like chocolate and whole raw milk cheese; lifestyle choices like sleeping late and laughing a lot; and downright shocking practices like going to the doctor less, taking fewer medications, and avoiding many prescribed but often unnecessary medical procedures. Seeing that these studies were in line with his own observations, Dr. Ofgang suggested that some of his patients continue to enjoy certain foods and lifestyle choices heretofore considered vices. This book grew from the idea that some of the foods and behaviors considered vices were actually "good vices."

Dr. Ofgang first came to admire some of these good vices while studying medicine in Italy. Here he gained an appreciation for what Italians call *la dolce vita*, "the sweet life," which can be described as consuming great food and fine drink, all in moderation and rarely to excess, surrounded by friends and family. Dr. Ofgang brought this appreciation back home to the United

States, and the Ofgang household was the site of home-brewed beer, home-milled whole grains, handmade pasta, fresh-baked bread, home-roasted coffee, and natural medicines.

Growing up within this context, Erik was equally fascinated with these pursuits and became a journalist and college professor focused on food and healthy living. One of his previous books is about beer and other craft beverages, and he is a professional food reviewer and health and science writer.

At first our discussions of the good vices were informal and fueled by our mutual love of many of them and our interest in the way healthy living often seems to coincide with happy living. When we decided to write about some of these vices, what started out as a fun collaboration for a short article turned into a much longer work. It sometimes was shocking to find that a lot of these vices, including playing in dirt and being exposed to certain bacteria, actually could make us healthier.

In the pages that follow, you'll be taken on a tour of many of these vices, and research supporting their possible health benefits will be presented alongside our own observations. You can read the book cover to cover, or pick and choose the vices that interest you the most. Along the way you'll see that we use the word *moderation* again and again. This caveat is important, as the secret to many of the good vices is enjoying them in moderation. For example, while moderate beer drinking may be healthy, excessive beer drinking is definitely not.

If you come across a vice that you don't already engage in, do not start it for health reasons; that is not the point of this book. We don't necessarily understand the reasons some of these good vices can be good for us; it's possible the joy we get from them is partly what makes them healthy.

As we explore the good vices, we will also keep an eye out for the way statistics and studies can be used to market and promote rather than educate and enlighten.

Often medical statistics are presented as relative statistics, which compare the odds of something happening for two groups in relation to each other. They are frequently confused with absolute statistics, which are the overall odds of something happening. Presenting only the relative statistics can make a treatment seem far more significant than it really is. Here's a real-world example of relative stats in action. Routine mammograms are often cited as providing women with a 20 percent decreased risk of death. On the surface, this sounds like an enormous benefit. However, since the 20 percent refers to relative, not absolute risk, the absolute difference between those who get mammogram screenings and those who do not is much, much smaller. One famous study in *The Lancet* found that out of 129,750 women who had mammograms, 511 died of breast cancer over the next fifteen years, a death rate of 0.4 percent. A different group of 117,260 women, who didn't have screenings, had 584 breast cancer deaths over the same time period, a death rate of 0.5 percent. That difference of one-tenth of 1 percent is what is used to declare the 20 percent improvement.[3] You can argue that the 0.1 percentage point improvement still is an improvement, and it is. It's just nowhere near the slam dunk it appears to be when a 20 percent improvement is mentioned. As Mark Twain said, "There are three kinds of lies: lies, damned lies, and statistics."

And these framed-in-a-good-light statistics may not be

accurate to begin with. One important study conducted by researchers at Beth Israel Medical Center in New York found favorable outcomes were significantly more common in studies sponsored by the drug manufacturer than in studies sponsored by a competitor or studies without pharmaceutical industry sponsorship. When the drug manufacturer sponsored a study looking at its own drug, it found favorable results 78 percent of the time; competitors found favorable outcomes only 28 percent of the time; and non-industry-sponsored studies found favorable outcomes 48 percent of the time.[4]

Conflicts of interest in health care are such that a 2009 report by the National Academy of Sciences, sponsored by the National Institutes of Health, found:

- Gifts from drug companies to physicians are ubiquitous.

- Visits to physicians' offices by drug and medical device company representatives and the provision of drug samples are widespread.

- Many faculty members receive research support from the pharmaceutical industry, which funds most of the biomedical research in the United States.

- Many faculty members and community physicians provide scientific, marketing, and other consulting services to companies; and some serve on company boards of directors or on industry speakers bureaus.

- Commercial sources provide about half of the total funding for accredited continuing medical education programs.

Recognizing that this was a problem, the authors of the report created a detailed set of recommendations to decrease the preponderance of conflict-of-interest issues "infecting" medical studies. These recommendations included calls to standardize stricter and more far-reaching disclosure statements and to reform physician interactions and financial links with the pharmaceutical industry, among many other efforts.[5]

Almost a decade later, little progress has been made on this front. Well-respected medical reviewers such as Cochrane have questioned the usefulness and the need for common procedures and so-called preventative measures like routine mammograms.[6,7] Research suggests that doctors who own their own MRI machines are more likely to order more MRIs, even for patients who may not need them.[8] A landmark study found people with osteoarthritis improved equally well regardless of whether they received a real surgical procedure (i.e., arthroscopic knee surgery) or a fake one (i.e., a placebo procedure).[9] Studies also show that commonly prescribed drugs like antibiotics,[10] antidepressants,[11,12] and antianxiety medications are often prescribed incorrectly, don't cure, or are overprescribed. In addition, the United States is alone among developed countries in its common practice of prophylactically administering antibiotic eye drops to newborns within an hour of birth. The treatment is supposed to prevent pinkeye caused by the sexually transmitted diseases gonorrhea and chlamydia present in the mother, but is a curious practice for children of mothers who have been screened during pregnancy and don't have either condition. Also, many of the antibiotics in use don't work on both diseases, and the eye drops are sometimes administered to babies that have been born via cesarean section, when the risk (which is virtually nonexistent anyhow) only theoretically applies to babies born vaginally.

Speaking of cesarean sections, as others have noted, "America's Caesarean rate includes over one-third of birthing women. This rate varies by state and ranges from 23% to 40%. This is nearly triple the World Health Organization's recommendation."[13]

All this leads us to caution the patient. Not only should the buyer (the patient) beware, but they should question their caregivers and do research on their own because the system has more than minor problems; in many ways it is broken. We tell you this not to upset you or to make you distrust all studies and medical professionals, but to encourage you to approach medicine with a healthy dose (pun intended) of skepticism, and that goes for the information offered in this book as well.

Remember, although this book is based on decades of experience and the best available research, it is not intended, and should not be taken, as medical advice. It does attempt to entertain and promote free, open-minded, kind, and diverse thought.

Health books deal in generalizations, but health is specific to each individual; and health-care, diet, and exercise decisions should be made in consultation with your health provider. In addition, new studies are constantly being conducted, and our understanding of what may or may not be healthy is always evolving.

Finally, though this book celebrates good vices, it is by no means advocating wanton hedonism. Our point is not to encourage people to eat and drink bad foods and smoke and gain weight. The point is for people to be happier and healthier by being freer and following truth. Alas, not every vice is good for us; your parents were right about the wisdom of avoiding many of them. Cigarettes are as bad for you as your mother told you they were. A little sugar may be fine, but excessive consumption of candy and sweets shouldn't be part of your daily routine, and bacon, we're sorry to say, appears to be good only for your soul.

But there are plenty of good vices, which aren't really vices at all because in moderation they can provide long-term enjoyment for the mind and body. We regularly tell patients that no matter how busy or stressed they are, they should do something that they look forward to each day. It can be a short walk with the dog, a quick bike ride or swim, a delicious dinner, a quick game of poker or blackjack, or a single malt scotch or cold beer. Even if we haven't discovered the "meaning of life," when we look forward to something each day, it gives that day a little bit more meaning.

When he was over seventy, the late great comedian Rodney Dangerfield told an audience that he had just come from his doctor, who told him that if he ate right, exercised, and got plenty of fresh air, he'd get old, sick, and die.

Too true.

Our fate is set and as far as we know, no one avoids leaving the earth when the time comes. What we want to do and can do is to have fun, live well, enjoy ourselves, and share health and happiness the best we can, for as long as we can.

If we stretch our time on earth a little longer and live a little better, all the better.

This book is a humble and lighthearted attempt to stack the

deck in your favor. We do this not by making life more rigid, restrictive, and boring, but more colorful, enjoyable, and fulfilling.

So get ready to learn about the benefits of a more satisfying, fun, and yes, healthier way of living. As they say in New Orleans: *Laissez les bons temps rouler,* or let the good times roll!

CHAPTER ONE

A BEER A DAY JUST MIGHT HELP KEEP THE DOCTOR AWAY

■ ■ ■

Beer he drank—seven goblets . . .
His heart was glad and his face shone.
—THE EPIC OF GILGAMESH, 2100 BC

IN BRIEF: Moderate beer drinking is a fun and healthy way to enjoy life. Approximately one glass of beer a day for men or women can have a plethora of health benefits, including a reduced risk of heart attacks and other cardiac events and type 2 diabetes.

It was time to set some things in stone.

Almost four thousand years ago, Hammurabi, the sixth king of Babylon, decided someone had to start keeping track of the rules. Around 1754 BC, he ordered what would become known as the Code of Hammurabi etched in a stone tablet. The revolutionary code was one of the first sets of written laws and contained more than 282 rules covering many aspects of human life and inspiring the "eye for an eye" justice later echoed in the Bible.

The code also addressed something less likely to be covered in your ancient history class: beer. Four laws within it govern the brewing and sale of beer, making it crystal clear where ancient society's priorities were.

In the nearly four millennia since these laws were literally set in stone, these priorities have not changed; beer is still one of the granddaddies of all vices, the companion many of us long for most deeply after a hard day's work. And in this instance, at least, our longings do not lead us astray. Beer, we are happy to report, not only tastes good, it is good for us, according to the research. In fact, when drunk in moderation, it appears beer may be really, really good for us.

As the Harvard School of Public Health recounted in an on-line analysis of alcohol's potential health benefits, "More than 100 prospective studies show an inverse association between moderate drinking and risk of heart attack, ischemic (clot-caused) stroke, peripheral vascular disease, sudden cardiac death, and death from all cardiovascular causes. The effect is fairly consistent, corresponding to a 25 percent to 40 percent reduction in risk."[1] (Take that, spinach!)

But what exactly constitutes moderate drinking?

We pondered this question over a couple of local craft beers at a brewery in Connecticut one stormy afternoon. We started happy hour early and were trying a sour beer, an ancient tart style of beer made with wild, naturally occurring yeast and lactobacillus, the same healthy bacteria used to sour yogurt.

The Centers for Disease Control and Prevention and most research define moderate drinking as about a drink or so a day for men and up to one drink a day for women. This drinking must be spread out; there's no skipping days in order to save up for a seven-drink bender on the weekend. In technical terms, a drink consists of 12 ounces of beer (an average-size can) with 5 percent alcohol content, 8 ounces of beer with 7 percent or higher alcohol content, 5 ounces of wine, or 1½ ounces (a shot) of hard liquor.[2]

A drink or so of this size may not result in epic stories of late nights spent dancing on top of bars, but it would be hard for even the most enthusiastic beer drinker to describe a beer each day as anything approaching abstinence. While keg stands and beer funnels are not part of the healthy living equation, there appears to be ample room in a healthy and happy life for a cold one after work or for enjoying a pint or two at a brewery or bar while talking with friends and family. Beer, we firmly believe, is something to look forward to, to savor and enjoy, not a substance to be sucked into the body at the quickest speed possible, as if you're a race car fueling up at a pit stop.

The beer we were drinking that afternoon was aged for months in large oak barrels where the wild yeast and lactobacillus worked their magic on the developing brew—ultimately creating an intense beer that demanded to be noticed. It had unusual earthy flavors and bright notes reminiscent of lemon and champagne that danced upon our taste buds.

In general, unfiltered beer made with locally grown organic hops is best. In laboratory studies, hop compounds have decreased cognitive decline and the chances of developing prostate and breast cancer.[3,4,5]

But not everyone takes this type of advice sitting down. Many years ago, a woman we were treating at our health center, Hahnemann Health, improved so much using the natural medicine approach that she forced her husband, who was something of a skeptic concerning natural health, to come in for an appointment. The husband wanted to know if there were any studies showing that *anything* natural helped to make you healthier. We told him, "Yes, possibly if you have a beer or so on most days, you might be healthier and happier and may even live longer."

He said, "What?!" and ran out of the office into the waiting room. We were afraid we had upset him, but a moment later he returned and said, "Please repeat that for my wife."

In 1990, an American Cancer Society study that examined the health of 275,000 men since 1959 found those who consumed one to two drinks a day had a mortality rate from coronary heart disease and all other causes significantly lower than those who never drank. (Though many studies have gotten similar results, there are also studies that contradict these findings, so drinkers beware.)

Once again, moderation is the key. In ancient days, the penalty for violating Hammurabi's beer-related laws—which included a rule against overcharging a patron—was death by drowning. Evidently Hammurabi *really* did not like expensive beer. According to some accounts, the "guilty" party would be drowned in a vat of beer; it was a powerful, if gruesome, reminder that sometimes you can have too much of a good thing. The American Cancer Society study offers the same lesson: Participants who consumed three or more drinks a day still had a lower risk of death from coronary heart disease, but they had a higher mortality rate overall.[6]

More recent research has resulted in similar findings. In fact, one could easily design a drinking game where you have a swig of beer every time you come across a study that espouses the benefits of moderate drinking. The only problem is that after a half hour of research, you will no longer be drinking moderately!

A 2004 study that surveyed 6,644 men and 8,010 women, age twenty-five to ninety-eight, concluded that people who drank about one drink a day on average had the "lowest all-cause mortality"— lower than those who had more than two drinks a day and lower than nondrinkers.[7]

A study published in the *American Journal of Epidemiology* analyzed results from 4,272 men and 1,761 women and found that those who reported having at least one drink a week were "significantly less likely to have poor cognitive function." These cognitive benefits extended even to those who had about thirty drinks a week, though at that level, the negative side effects outweigh the positives.[8] Another study conducted by researchers at the Harvard T. H. Chan School of Public Health looked at 38,031 middle-aged American men and found that participants who rarely drank could reduce their risk of type 2 diabetes by increasing their alcohol intake to one or two drinks a day.[9]

We could keep going, but we think you get the point: Beer's healthy properties have been widely recognized in scores of studies. So just in case you are playing that drinking game, we're going to stop here.

Surprising as it is, the fact that beer and other alcoholic beverages have some health benefits makes sense from a biological standpoint. Drinking in moderation raises levels of high-density lipoprotein (HDL, or "good" cholesterol), which is associated with protection against heart disease. It is possible this is why alcohol has been linked to decreased blood clotting, which causes fewer blocked arteries and therefore strokes.

Beyond the benefits that all alcohol seems to offer, beer contains antioxidants, cancer fighters, and immune enhancers unique to the malt- and hop-powered beverage. Researchers at Oregon State University have studied a compound within hops—an integral ingredient that gives beer its bitter flavor and strong aroma—that has cancer-fighting abilities[10] and has been shown in the laboratory setting to lower cholesterol and blood sugar and help with weight loss in animals.[11] In addition, the yeast that powers beer's fermentation process, turning sugar into alcohol, has a positive immune effect.

In 2011, researchers at Italy's Fondazione di Ricerca e Cura analyzed data from more than 100,000 people and concluded that those who drank a pint of beer a day had a 31 percent lower risk of heart disease compared to nondrinkers.[12]

That's not to say all the news regarding drinking beer and other alcohol is good. This is earth, after all, not heaven. Excessive drinking is unhealthy and the risk of addiction is real. Women, in particular, should be aware of potential adverse effects. Some research suggests that even moderate alcohol consumption can cause increased risks of breast cancer. A 2014 review of epidemiologic and experimental studies looking at alcohol's links to breast cancers concluded that each additional drink a woman consumes per day increases the relative risk (the comparison of risk between two groups) of breast cancer, but not the absolute risk (the overall risk of developing a given disease people in the general population have).[13]

The negative effects of beer and other alcohol could be caused by the fact that they block the body's absorption of folate, the B vitamin that helps to build our DNA and is essential for accurate cell divisions in our bodies. It is possible that some of the ill effects of alcohol in women can be mitigated by increasing one's intake of folate—either by eating foods rich in the vitamin, like black beans, lentils, and dark greens including spinach, lettuce, and asparagus, or by taking B vitamins. A study of 88,818 women found that among drinkers of one or more alcoholic drinks a day, moderate drinkers with higher levels of folate in their blood were 90 percent less likely to develop breast cancer than drinkers who had the lowest levels of folate.[14]

Based on this and other studies, some experts believe an intake of folate of at least 600 micrograms a day can mitigate some of the negative effects of alcohol consumption.

We are not here to promote drinking, especially excessive drinking. On the contrary, as with other vices in this book, we encourage the middle road of moderation and common sense. Having said that, many studies show a drink a day may actually be beneficial. There are, of course, studies that dispute this. For example, a recent major study appearing in *The Lancet* came to the literally sobering conclusion that drinking any alcohol, even moderate amounts, is detrimental to health.[15] The study focused on relative, not absolute, risk and seemingly contradicted many other studies, including one published just a few months before in *The Lancet*. As David Spiegelhalter, the Winton Professor for the

Public Understanding of Risk at the University of Cambridge, noted, one figure in the appendix of the earlier study showed "that, compared to moderate drinkers, 'never-drinkers' experience 30% more heart disease and strokes, and 20% higher overall death rate. But this does not mean that this is because they don't drink."[16]

Another question the new study leaves unanswered is why residents of certain European countries have a higher life expectancy even though they drink more than in the United States. There could be many reasons for this discrepancy beyond alcohol's health effects, but either way, it warrants further study. Even if you accept the premise of risk in the study, at the low levels of alcohol consumption we discussed, the absolute risk associated with low to moderate consumption is extremely low. We always recommend seeing both sides with an open mind and suggest taking this (and many studies) with a grain of salt in one hand and a glass of unfiltered beer in the other.

The CDC does not recommend that nondrinkers start drinking for health, although the agency doesn't tell those who already drink moderately for fun to stop. And the dietary guidelines provided by the U.S. Department of Health between 2015 and 2020 allow for the drinking of one to two drinks a day for men and one drink a day for women (although it's possible the CDC will recommend decreased amounts based on new studies in the future).

Remember that as the Harvard T. H. Chan School of Public Health points out, "The definition of moderate drinking is something of a balancing act. Moderate drinking sits at the point at which the health benefits of alcohol clearly outweigh the risks."[17]

As we drank the sour beer at the brewery in Connecticut, we were reminded that more than 3,500 years after Hammurabi's Code originated, beer remains an important part of most modern societies, and with all it brings to the table healthwise and otherwise, we're thankful it still is. In memory of Hammurabi, we propose a drink both to and for your health.

CHAPTER TWO

WINE, WINE, SO VERY FINE

■ ■ ■

A man cannot make him laugh;
but that's no marvel, he drinks no wine.
—WILLIAM SHAKESPEARE, *HENRY IV*

IN BRIEF: Like beer, moderate wine drinking is a fun and healthy way to enjoy life. Approximately one glass of wine per day for men or women can have many health benefits, including a reduced risk of heart attacks and other cardiac events and type 2 diabetes.

In Victor Hugo's *Les Misérables,* Jean Valjean is sentenced to five years' imprisonment for stealing bread to feed his starving family. Thanks to the draconian legal system of 1800s France, this five-year sentence stretches to nineteen years. During that time Valjean is forced to work the oars in the galleys of French ships and is locked in the Bagne of Toulon, an infamous dungeon-like prison. Here, Valjean and his real-world counterparts have an iron ring and chain weighing about fifteen pounds clasped around their ankles. Along with meager daily portions of bread and bean soup, they received a daily ration of wine . . . yes, wine.

At the time, it was acceptable to jail people for years for a minor infraction, chain them to their beds by night, and force them into hellish, terrifying labor by day, but deprive them of wine? You can't do that.

That would be cruel.

Today the galleys are long gone, but wine remains as much a part of French culture as cheese, frog legs, and hard-to-pronounce words. The beverage's considerable health benefits, and the healthy appetite those living in France have for it, often are thought to contribute to the "French Paradox," the counterintuitive way in which the French have lower rates of coronary heart disease while enjoying a diet high in saturated fats.

Indeed, when it comes to possible medicinal alcohol consumption, wine is in many ways the poster child of healthy drinking. Its potential health benefits have been recognized longer and are met with less skepticism than the benefits of beer or spirits.

Wine drinkers, like alcohol drinkers in general, enjoy a wide variety of benefits above and beyond the flavor of their drink of choice. More than a hundred studies point to between a 25 and 40 percent reduction in risk of death from all cardiovascular causes for moderate wine drinkers. The beverage also has been linked to decreased rates of type 2 diabetes and slower cognitive decline. Just remember, as with beer, these benefits have been found in moderate drinkers: those who drink about one or so 5-ounce glasses of wine a day.[1]

We're halfway through our first 5-ounce glass of wine for the day at an Italian restaurant a short drive from New York City. We discuss how in addition to the general positive effects of moderate alcohol consumption, wine has many unique health properties and is rich in antioxidants and nutrients. Some of the world's longest-living people consume it regularly. In *The Blue Zones,* author Dan Buettner discusses the lifestyle traits of centenarians, people a hundred years old and older, in areas of the world where there are extremely large numbers of them. For example, in Sardinia, Italy, where there are ten times more centenarians per capita than in the United States, Buettner and his fellow researchers found long-lived Sardinians generally walked several miles a day throughout their lives, ate a mostly plant-based diet with occasional meat, were deeply connected to their communities and families, and enjoyed a glass or two of wine daily.

These aged Sardinians would find much to enjoy at this restaurant. It's family owned and operated, and each meal is prepared fresh with great care. The portions are medium sized, and sauces are used sparingly, but are rich with flavor. The wine is important, but not *the* most important part of the meal; that honor belongs to the food itself and to the sense of companionship shared by those dining.

In the 1970s, the elder of this book's coauthors was a medical student in Italy, and it was then that he first witnessed the cultured and moderate appreciation of wine that Buettner observed in the Sardinians. Harry lived in a beautiful city where the ancient stone street was shaded by medieval archways, with a central piazza that was a beacon for the community.

It was here that, as noted in the introduction, Harry came to appreciate what Italians call *la dolce vita,* "the sweet life." He would unwind after long days studying medical textbooks with a glass or two (okay, sometimes more) of the local vintage at home or with friends in town, often while enjoying handmade pasta and other Italian delicacies.

Almost every farm had grapes, and farmers made their own wine. Many of these wines were stored in giant roadside containers reminiscent of propane tanks. The wine could be purchased at bargain prices and you'd bring your own 50-liter demijohn and have it filled, much like one might buy gas here.

Harry also gained an appreciation of the hard work that went into harvesting the grapes for wine after working as a grape picker for a local vineyard in Umbria, Italy. Picking grapes was difficult, stooped labor. The more seasoned farmworkers (*contadini*) at the vineyard taught him to conserve energy by slowing down when the owner (*padrone*) was not around. When the landlord was nearby, cries of "*Il padrone!*" would ring out in warning from other grape pickers, so all of them could pick up the pace a bit and avoid any trouble. The lesson of these temporary slowdowns was that hard work and relaxation are not diametrically opposed, and that at the end of a long day in the fields picking grapes, one could, and arguably should, treat oneself to the fruit of that labor.

In Connecticut in the present day, as our meal draws to a close, Patty Ofgang (Harry's wife and Erik's mother) recalls how in Italy, the appreciation of wine extends from the countryside into medical facilities. She worked as a nurse at an Italian hospital, where her duties included giving each patient their daily allotment of wine. She says that quite often, this and some chamomile tea would make it unnecessary to give a patient a sleeping pill in the evening. She and Harry fondly recall the oft-heard chant by young and old alike in Italy: *"L'acqua fa male, il vino fa cantare"* (water makes you feel bad, wine makes you sing).

The concept of wine in hospitals may be alien to many, but wine as medicine has a long history. Hippocrates, who was born in 460 BC, used wine as a disinfectant to clean wounds, mixed it with herbs to make them more palatable, and used it as medicine in its own right—prescribing the drink as a cure for diarrhea and pain during childbirth. He once wrote, "Wine is an appropriate article for mankind, both for the healthy body and for the ailing man."

Moderate wine drinking by those who treat wine not as a highway to drunkenness but as an ingredient in *la dolce vita*, to relax from the hustle and bustle of daily life, may bring not only the momentary delight of the wine but also may help the drinker live longer and age more gracefully.

The evidence has long supported these observations, and the studies highlighting wine's many virtues continue to be conducted. In 2015, the *Annals of Internal Medicine* published a study in which participants in Israel with controlled type 2 diabetes were randomly assigned to drink either 150 milliliters (a little more than 5 ounces) of mineral water, white wine, or red wine with dinner for two years. All three groups followed a Mediterranean diet without caloric restriction.

The results give red wine lovers plenty to toast.

Those assigned to drink red wine saw modest but significant decreases in cardiometabolic risk (a person's chances of having diabetes, heart disease, or stroke), in part because it increased HDL (good cholesterol). As an added bonus, drinkers of both red and white wine enjoyed better-quality sleep than the water drinkers. Unlike many alcohol studies, which are epidemiology studies, this was a randomized control study, considered a better method for pinpointing specific traits or behaviors.[2]

A 2005 study published in *The American Journal of Gastroenterology* found that those who had one to eight glasses of wine a week were less likely to develop colon tumors.[3] And wine, like beer and spirits, has been shown to reduce cognitive decline and the onset of Alzheimer's, as well as decrease the chances of developing type 2 diabetes.[4]

In particular, two ingredients in wine are hailed for their health-giving properties: resveratrol and procyanidins. Resveratrol is a naturally occurring compound found in grape skins that has been linked to reductions in osteoporosis, decreased fat cell production, and reduction of blood pressure. Particularly prevalent in red wine, resveratrol has been shown to slow the aging-related degenerative process in the lungs of mice[5] and increase the lifespan of mice on high-calorie diets.[6]

As incredible as some of these laboratory results on resveratrol have been, a 2006 study by researchers at Queen Mary, University of London, concluded that there was not enough resveratrol present in wine to account for the beverage's health benefits. Instead, this study suggested that procyanidin compounds, also found in wine, are more likely responsible for some of wine's health benefits. They found procyanidins "are present at higher concentrations in wines from areas of southwestern France and Sardinia, where traditional production methods ensure that these compounds are efficiently extracted during vinification." As the study concluded,

"These regions also happen to be associated with increased longevity in the population."[7]

Despite the unique health properties of wine, recent studies have suggested the health benefits of wine, beer, and spirits are more closely related. In other words, wine's healthiest ingredients are not fully understood. If you're a wine drinker, cheers and keep on drinking what you're drinking. If you're a beer or spirits drinker, there's not enough evidence showing a significant difference between wine and other alcoholic beverages to justify an unwanted switch, though it never hurts to broaden your drinking horizons, so mix in a glass of wine here and there.[8]

As with beer and other alcohol, drinking wine may have some risk, especially for women, but overall many negative studies are inconclusive and at this point indicate that the rewards of moderate drinking may outweigh the risks.

Whether you're locked up in a French dungeon like Jean Valjean or find yourself in an Italian hospital, wine—the drink of both peasants and kings—may be a good dietary choice and is a key part of the lifestyle of many of the globe's healthiest cultures and communities. As those who live on the Mediterranean are already aware, wine can be an important part of living *la dolce vita*.

CHAPTER THREE

MOVED BY THE SPIRITS

■ ■ ■

For all things good, mezcal.
For all things bad as well.
—ANONYMOUS

IN BRIEF: Those who drink approximately one shot of gin, vodka, tequila, whiskey, cognac, or other spirits a day seem to enjoy similar benefits as wine and beer drinkers. This may include a decrease in the chance of death from all cardiovascular causes. Avoid sugary mixed drinks and focus on forming enjoyable rituals around your alcohol consumption, like meeting with friends or relaxing after work.

While in his early nineties, Nathan "Nussie" Ofgang, the father and grandfather of Harry and Erik, respectively, visited his cardiologist's office in West Palm Beach, Florida. As the specialist began his examination, he asked Nussie who had driven him, a routine question for patients his age.

"I drove myself," he said with the friendly-but-to-the-point vintage New York attitude that had been forged nearly a century earlier on the streets of Brownsville in Brooklyn.

"Who does your shopping?" the cardiologist asked.

"I do my shopping."

"Who cooks dinner for you?"

"I do."

After confirming with a few more questions that Nussie was indeed extremely active and fully independent, the cardiologist said, "Go home, I'll see you in six months. You should be giving me advice."

It was a story that Nussie was fond of repeating to his children and grandchildren. When anyone asked what the secret to his long and healthy life was, he remarked: "I don't sit on my ass at a computer all day like most young people [i.e., everyone under ninety]. I keep busy. I eat a lot of garlic and onions *and* I drink a glass of scotch every day."

This glass of scotch wasn't the only factor in his longevity, and he didn't actually begin sipping the water of life daily until retirement, but whiskey, like other alcoholic drinks when enjoyed in moderation, may be something of a health tonic. As we've noted in the chapters on beer and wine, dozens of studies have shown moderate drinking decreases the chance of death from all cardiovascular causes by 25 to 40 percent. For spirits—defined as a distilled drink with a 20 percent ABV (alcohol by volume) or higher—a moderate amount means about a drink or so, with a drink being 1½ ounces or about one shot.[1]

Moderate consumption of spirits, like other alcohol, raises our bodies' levels of high-density lipoprotein (HDL, or "good" cholesterol), which, as previously noted, has been associated with protection against heart disease.

Alcohol also can be an effective painkiller. Analyzing eighteen studies and looking at 404 people, researchers at London's

University of Greenwich found that alcohol can provide more effective pain relief than Tylenol. The study concluded that those with a mean blood alcohol content of about .08 percent, the amount reached after three to four drinks, enjoyed a "moderate to large reduction in pain intensity ratings." In fact, the pain reductions offered by alcohol were comparable to that of opioids. Three to four drinks of beer, wine, or booze is more than we recommend drinking daily, but alcohol's pain-reducing effects are definitely worth toasting.[2]

The potential health benefits of various spirits have long been noted. The ancient Latin term for whiskey was *aqua vitae,* water of life. In the seventeenth century, gin, a distilled spirit flavored with juniper berries, anise, caraway, coriander, and other botanicals, was sold in Dutch pharmacies to treat a variety of medical ailments including kidney problems, stomach problems, gallstones, and gout. We wouldn't recommend treating these ailments today with nothing more than a glass of gin on the rocks, but distilled beverages may offer some surprising benefits.

For a study published in the journal *Consciousness and Cognition,* researchers at the University of Illinois at Chicago split forty young men into two groups. One group watched a movie and was served vodka cranberry drinks until their blood alcohol level was brought up to .75 percent, just below the legal driving limit of .80 percent. The other group watched a movie but did not drink alcohol. Both groups took a mental acuity test. Surprisingly, the drinking group solved more problems in less time and was "more likely to perceive their solutions as the result of a sudden insight."

The sample size of this experiment was small, so we can't draw too large a conclusion here, but the study was built on previous research indicating that forgetfulness can help us think more creatively. A lack of concentration, or selectively poor memory, could allow people to be less burdened by precedent and therefore more open to innovative ideas. Alcohol *might* be a way to get to this productively forgetful state, as the authors conclude: The study supports "earlier suggestions that creative problem solving may benefit from a more diffuse attentional state and shows that moderate intoxication may be one way to alter attentional states to be more conducive to creative processing."[3]

Booze, counterintuitively, has even been shown in some studies to help in the bedroom. In a survey of more than one thousand men, researchers in Australia found that compared with those who never drank, chances of erectile dysfunction were lower "among current, weekend and binge drinkers." In fact, drinkers in the study were 25 to 30 percent less likely than their nondrinking counterparts to develop the condition that has become a punch line thanks to far too many commercials advertising drugs that treat it. Yes, the sample size was small, but it did contain, shall we say, some hard evidence.[4]

In order to be healthy while you drink, always be mindful of what type of alcohol you consume. Many mixed drinks at restaurants and bars are essentially sugar-filled hangover potions made with bottom-shelf, off-label products. As any small-batch craft distiller will tell you, low-quality alcohol is distilled with less care and often contains higher quantities of non-ethanol alcohol, which our bodies have trouble processing and are thought to be more likely to cause headaches. Fortunately, there are many new craft distilleries opening up across the United States, and there remain high-quality spirit producers in Europe, Mexico, and elsewhere with products that, when drunk in moderation, will not cause hangovers and have rich enough flavors that it's not necessary to obscure them with sugary cocktail mixes. A good rule of thumb, both to avoid hangovers and high-calorie mixed drinks, is that if you're not sure if what you're drinking is actually a high-quality distilled spirit, don't drink it.

Recently, an old family friend of ours, a lifelong nondrinker who also happens to be a leading authority on statistics, became so convinced of alcohol's health benefits that he began drinking for medical reasons. During our annual Super Bowl party, he made a minor scene when as the clock struck seven, he pulled out a shot-sized bottle of whiskey, and with all the joy of a four-year-old being forced to eat broccoli, drank it with palpable distaste.

Unlike other guests at the party, who were drinking for fun as they watched the game, he drank his daily "dose" of alcohol in the exact same manner he took medication. He may have gotten some benefits from alcohol consumption with this method, but he was missing the bigger picture, and we don't believe he was doing himself many favors in the long run. In any case, imbibing alcohol as he would take medicine proved unsustainable for him, and he gave it up within a few months.

Alcohol is not cough syrup and shouldn't be treated like blood pressure medication. For those who already enjoy it, it can be a powerful tonic, but we believe it has the strongest effect on our health and well-being when it is used as part of the equation for a healthy and happy life—when we drink for enjoyment and friendship.

Despite our passion for spirits and what can be done with them, we do not engage in nor advocate excessive drinking. You're better off drinking less and savoring something that is of higher quality. When someone is sipping the finest of the fine spirits—like Islay Single Malt Scotch, which has been aging in barrels for many years, or handmade mezcal, lovingly distilled from rare wild agave plants—it's almost as if the artistry and zest for life bestowed by the master craftsmen are somehow infused into the individual. Like alchemy, the more carefully crafted alcohols, liquors, and spirits have a kind of hidden magical benefit of transforming the spirit of the individual, not just physically, but also mentally and emotionally.

Grandpa Nussie drank scotch with the reverence that some cultures display in ancestor worship, and the joy with which one witnesses a sunset in summer. He was one of the hardest-working men we'd ever met. He grew up during the Great Depression and became his family's main financial provider as a teenager. After marrying and serving in the Navy during World War II, he bought a vending machine business. To support his family, he claimed, with only slight exaggeration, he worked 24/7 for seven years. His little sleep was often punctuated by calls for repairs at restaurants, gin mills (bars), and hotels in the middle of the night. In order to spend time with his young children, he frequently took them to work with him, traversing the length and breadth of New York City.

Years later, when he had retired to Florida, he had little desire to stop working. During visits, we would marvel at how in his nineties, he had the energy to wake well before dawn each morning, make his coffee, sharpen his cooking knives, and clean his stove with a toothbrush. Then while it was still dark, he'd head to one of his many volunteer jobs. He was a chef at a soup kitchen, worked as a set builder at a local playhouse, served as a volunteer sheriff, and also worked in the pharmacy and infectious disease unit of a local hospital. This hospital even would call him in to brief new pharmacists.

But no matter how hard he pushed himself during the day, four P.M. was quitting time. The hard work he had engaged in would be shed as he sat for a half hour to an hour with a favorite glass of scotch, listening to classical music and reading a book. For a man who generally didn't like to relax, he achieved a near-meditative state of calm during this time. It was his personal cocktail hour, and nothing and no one could interfere with that.

This is the way to enjoy spirits, as part of a ritual that you look forward to and that improves your overall well-being. Grandpa Nussie may have started an hour before the traditional cocktail hour, but as many signs in his Florida neighborhood proudly proclaimed with a Zen-like wisdom not normally found on barroom doors outside of Margaritaville: *It's Five O'Clock Somewhere. Sláinte* and *L'chaim* (To your health)!

CHAPTER FOUR

SLEEP

Life's Meditation

■ ■ ■

From breakfast on through all the day
At home among my friends I stay,
But every night I go abroad
Afar into the land of Nod.
—ROBERT LOUIS STEVENSON

A good laugh and a long sleep are the best cures
in the doctor's book.
—IRISH PROVERB

IN BRIEF: Not getting enough sleep has been linked to an increased incidence of cardiovascular disease, cancer, and weight gain. By getting more and better-quality sleep, and waking naturally without an alarm, not only will you be healthier, but you may also be more efficient, get more work done, and even lose more weight. And because you'll be more efficient, it should be okay to head to work or school a little later. (Well, it's okay with us, but it may not be with your boss or teacher.)

Sleeping is a sin. Or at least that's what the Puritan minister Cotton Mather argued in a 1700s sermon, "Vigilius. Or, The Awakener," while raging against those who sleep when they should be working instead.

Mather was not alone in his disdain for snoozing. U.S. founding father Benjamin Franklin said, "There'll be sleeping enough in the grave," and Edgar Allan Poe once wrote, "Sleep, those little slices of death—how I loathe them."

In today's world, the rhetoric around sleep has softened, but our attitude toward it hasn't necessarily changed. We still view it as the bedfellow of laziness, something to enjoy as infrequently as possible or a necessary evil.

Sleep may be the only undeniably healthy activity that we feel guilty about. We're racked with guilt if we sleep in on the weekend or don't get up early enough to be productive. But have we ever had similar thoughts about getting fresh air? Or eating too much broccoli?

Rarely do healthy people sleep excessively, so feeling bad about sleeping "too much" is equally absurd. It's like apologizing for calling your mother *too* often.

Sleep, despite the way our society often views it, is not a luxury—it's a necessity. Exactly why all humans and animals need sleep is unknown, but it is clear that when we don't get it, bad things happen. Short-term sleep deprivation causes decreased alertness and fatigue. Stay up for several days straight, and the body starts going haywire, with hallucinations likely. Remain awake long enough and you might die; extended sleep deprivation attempts are so dangerous that Guinness World Records does not track or monitor them.

Lack of sleep also wreaks long-term havoc on our bodies.

Chronic undersleepers put themselves at an increased risk for a variety of ailments, including type 2 diabetes,[1] cardiovascular disease,[2] and possibly increased occurrences of breast, prostate, and colorectal cancer.[3]

Many we talk to remain unfazed by these negative associations with sleep deprivation. "I get it," they say, "but I like to go out late," or "I need to wake up early for work." Then we tell them about another side effect of sleep deprivation, one that is far more terrifying to some than decreased longevity: weight gain.

One large analysis of 68,183 women in the Nurses' Health Study found women who slept five hours or less per night weighed an average of 4.71 pounds more than those who got seven hours or more of sleep a night, even after the numbers were adjusted for age. Over a sixteen-year period, the five-hours-a-night sleepers gained 2.51 pounds more than those who got more than seven hours. Women who slept only about six hours gained 1.56 pounds more than the solid seven-hour sleepers. These results were not affected by diet or exercise.[4]

If that isn't causing you to lose sleep about losing sleep, this probably will: A 2006 literature review of the link between lack of sleep and weight gain, coauthored by Frank B. Hu of the Harvard T. H. Chan School of Public Health, suggested that for children, "short sleep duration is strongly and consistently associated with concurrent and future obesity." For adults, seventeen of twenty-three studies supported "independent association between short sleep duration and increased weight."[5]

Despite our society's increasing recognition of sleep's importance, we seem to be getting less and less slumber. According to one study, between 1985 and 2012, the number of people in the United States who slept only 6 hours or less rose by 31 percent, while the average person's time spent sleeping shrunk from 7.40 hours a night to 7.18 hours a night.[6]

The good news is that by following our instincts and sleeping more, we can quickly improve our health. As the National Sleep Foundation puts it, sleep is "as important as diet and exercise, only easier."

You should sleep soundly and well for about eight hours. Then, ideally, wake up refreshed without being prompted by an alarm clock. Try to look forward to at least one special thing each day, whether it's a walk in the park, a home-cooked meal, a movie, golf, baseball, fishing, tea, espresso, chocolate, or whatever good vice you choose.

We recommend going to sleep earlier in the night when possible. There's an old belief we subscribe to that sleep before midnight is more effective than after. As we'll note in our chapter on sunshine, by allowing more sunlight into your bedroom in the morning and not shutting out the sun with window shades, we can put our bodies more in line with the natural day-and-night cycle of the earth and therefore sleep more soundly. Apparently the old adage "Early to bed and early to rise makes a man healthy, wealthy, and wise" might be true.

Although we include coffee in our list of "good vices," remember it's best to wake up naturally and not jolt yourself awake with any stimulant. So at least sometimes try to put off that first cup of joe for an hour or two after you wake up.

Many people don't get enough sleep not because they don't want to, but because they don't think they have enough time. But decreasing the amount one sleeps to increase productivity is as much a mistake as decreasing sleep to exercise.

We are at our best when we're well rested and not foggy from tiredness. Not only does sleep help clear toxins, but it also helps us process the day's events and increases our ability to solve complex problems. In a German study, participants were taught to solve a difficult math problem, but were not taught a simple method for quickly solving it. Participants were divided into two groups to be retested eight hours later on the problem; one group pulled an all-nighter studying for it, while the other group was allowed to sleep. The group that was well rested was twice as likely to find the quicker solution.[7]

If you don't get enough sleep, try napping. Even a few minutes can be helpful, though generally it is best to keep naps shorter than an hour to avoid grogginess.

Dr. Henry Lindlahr, one of the founding fathers of naturopathic medicine, would teach the heads of state, industry leaders, and power brokers who came to his clinic from all over the world a technique whereby they would lightly hold a pencil between their fingers, close their eyes, and "steal" a few minutes of deep sleep right at their desks. They knew they had fallen into a deep sleep if the pencil dropped. (Don't try this if you've taken our advice elsewhere in this book and switched over to a standing desk.)

For a study published in *Nature Neuroscience*, researchers tested subjects on perceptual performances four times during the day. They found that the performance of those who did not nap deteriorated with each test, but those who took a thirty-minute nap between tests halted the deterioration, and those who took a sixty-minute nap reversed it.[8]

Naps also seem to improve the mood and memory of children, and there's a growing movement toward companies allowing employees to take naps while on the clock. One *New York Times* headline read: "Take Naps at Work. Apologize to No One."

Of course, not sleeping enough on occasion isn't necessarily unhealthy, and burning the midnight oil when needed is perfectly acceptable.

The U.S. Centers for Disease Control and Prevention (CDC) recommends at least seven hours of sleep for adults, with an hour or so more recommended for those over sixty, and between eight to ten hours of sleep for teenagers up to eighteen years old. The obstacles to getting this required sleep are many.

Getting nine hours of sleep can be all but impossible for teens because as a result of puberty, the teenage brain has trouble entering sleep mode before 10:45 P.M. Despite this late sleep time encouraged by their biology, most teenagers must wake up in time to be at school as early as 7:00 or 7:30 A.M.

There's a nationwide trend toward moving school district start times later, and the results are overwhelmingly positive. A 2014 multi-site study of 9,000 students found those enrolled in schools that started at 8:30 A.M. or later had improved grades and attendance, and decreased chances of substance abuse and symptoms of depression. In addition, the number of automobile crashes for teens between sixteen and eighteen years old was reduced by 70 percent; this statistic is significant because car accidents are the leading cause of death for teens in the United States, tragically claiming more than 2,000 young lives a year.[9]

In 2014, the American Academy of Pediatrics began to recommend delaying school start times until after 8:30 A.M., followed in 2016 by similar recommendations from the American Medical Association.[10,11]

Despite the clear health benefits, later school start times have met with fierce resistance. Critics point to logistical issues with school bus routes, and the move often is opposed by teachers who complain it will make their schedules worse.

Both criticisms could be easily resolved by a bold and, we think, innovative suggestion. How about a shorter workday or school day, and a shorter but more efficient workweek? We've seen no evidence that eight hours or six and a half hours are the optimal amounts of time for productivity at work or school. One trial in the city of Gothenburg in Sweden mandated a six-hour workday and a thirty-hour workweek. Officials in the city found employees completed as much or more work in the decreased time. In New Zealand, Perpetual Guardian, a business that manages trusts, tested the effect of having its employees work four days and thirty-two hours per week while getting paid for five days. They found employees took shorter breaks, were more motivated and creative, and concentrated on work while they were there—actually accomplishing more than they had in a traditional workweek.[12]

In any case, the criticism of later school start times pales in comparison to the emotional and physical health benefits of adolescents' being well rested and alert. In recent studies, schools that started their first class an hour later saw grades improve among their well-rested students, and schools that shortened the school week saw improvements as well. We bet companies would see similar improvements if the workday and workweek were shortened.

School and work aren't the only institutions waging war on the land of nod.

A lot of society is geared later than it should be. Many concerts don't start until after nine or ten P.M., and it's hard to find bars that are really hopping early in the evening. *Monday Night Football* and other major sporting events start too late for most kids to watch, and force adults to choose between watching their favorite sports team and being tired all the next day. Even baseball, our beloved national pastime, is sadly played *past* the healthy bedtime for most school-age kids and the rest of us.

While there's nothing you can do to get the first pitch of the World Series thrown earlier, you can make some changes on a personal level to improve your sleep. One easy step is to start limiting your use of cell phones and other exposure to LED screens before bedtime. The light from LED screens and lamps can suppress melatonin, the hormone that signals to the brain that it's time to sleep. One meta-analysis (a systematic review of the results of multiple previous studies) of more than 125,000 children found bedtime access to phones and other media devices was significantly associated with "inadequate sleep quantity, poor sleep quality, and excessive daytime sleepiness."[13]

Once you've turned off your LED lights and peeled your eyes from your phone, the next step you may want to consider is to throw out your pajamas and go au naturel for sleep. Sleeping naked might scare your roommates and houseguests, but it lowers body temperature and helps people fall asleep.

You also may want to get more sunlight. As we'll discuss later, one study found office workers in workspaces with more windows and natural sunlight enjoyed longer, better-quality sleep, had more positive outlooks, and engaged in more physical activity than those who worked in windowless offices. So try to get more sunlight during the day, regardless of what your workplace is like.[14]

If these tips don't work, sleeping pills are *most likely not* the answer. Sleeping pills, whether over-the-counter or prescription, generally increase total sleep time only between eleven and twenty-five minutes. Users often think the pills have helped more than they have because many sleeping pills make it harder for people to form memories. So if you take sleeping pills, it's theorized that you still may wake up in the night, but you're less likely to remember it. In addition, there are numerous possible side effects of sleeping pills, so it's better to eat right and exercise more to get a better-quality sleep.

Remember, practicing even one healthy habit tends to create a positive cycle by promoting and reinforcing other healthy behaviors. Getting good-quality sleep often means eating better, exercising more, decreasing stress, and having more fun and a more positive outlook. So by simply improving the quality of sleep, we are improving our general health as well.

More sleep is something you both want and need, so stop feeling guilty about it. If you come in late to work one day because you needed rest, instead of a doctor's note, give the boss a copy of this book with this chapter bookmarked. Odds are, he or she could use a little extra shut-eye as well.

CHAPTER FIVE

SEX, DRUGS, AND ROCK AND ROLL (OKAY, JUST SEX)

■ ■ ■

All you need is love.
—THE BEATLES

I spent half my money on gambling, alcohol,
and wild women. The other half I wasted.
—W. C. FIELDS

IN BRIEF: Sex is a great source of exercise and has been shown to help boost one's immune system, lower one's blood pressure and risk of heart disease, and improve one's mental and physical well-being. It also can help keep men's and women's levels of testosterone and estrogen in balance, and being in a committed, loving relationship can increase longevity for both men and women.

Throw out your nasal spray. According to the tried-and-true family periodical *Reader's Digest*, "Sex is reputedly a natural antihistamine, helping to combat hay fever and asthma symptoms." The same article reports that a Welsh study showed "the risk of dying in any one year was 50 percent lower among men who had sex twice or more a week than among men who had sex less than once a month. . . . The study concluded that the more sex, the better."[1]

Indeed, when it comes to the good vices covered in this book, sex is among the least complicated and most natural. It is enjoyable, beneficial to our health, and necessary to humanity's continued existence on this planet.

Many of us, regardless of what we might admit publicly, wouldn't mind having more sex. So you likely don't need any encouragement from us to pursue it, but in this chapter we'll tell you even more reasons you should be happy about enjoying it, and why you might want to consider making time for sex, no matter how busy your schedule is.

To begin with, love (i.e., lovemaking) literally is good for your heart.

One study found that men who had sex twice a week were 45 percent less likely to develop cardiovascular disease than men who had sex once a month or less.[2] Another study found men who had frequent orgasms were 50 percent less likely to die from all-cause mortality than those with infrequent orgasms.[3] Yet another research project concluded that men who had regular orgasms through conventional sex had lower blood pressure. Unfortunately for fans of the Internet's most popular "home videos," these effects did not translate to what we'll politely call "solo practitioners."[4]

And of course sex isn't just good for men. For women, sex can serve as a workout for pelvic muscles, helping to improve bladder control, thereby decreasing the chance of incontinence, which by some estimates affects 30 percent of women at some point during their lives.

It's also great exercise for everyone. As is true with other physical activities, sex raises the heart rate and strengthens muscles, but this pursuit, unlike running, is one that many of us actually look forward to. During sex men burn four calories per minute and women burn three calories per minute, a not-insignificant amount that certainly can add up.[5]

Sex also can supercharge the immune system. A study of 112 American college students found that those who had sex three or more times a week had significantly higher levels of immunoglobulin A (IgA)—an antibody that plays an important role in our immune system—than those who had sex twice a week or less. (No wonder people who never take sick days are more cheerful!)[6]

The act of lovemaking has been found to limit pain for both sexes. One study from 2013 suggested sex could help stop headaches—a somewhat ironic finding, since one of the classic reasons not to have sex throughout the ages has been the dreaded headache.[7]

During the act, serotonin, endorphins, and other feel-good hormones are released, limiting stress and creating feelings of elation that some credit with helping them fall asleep.

In what will come as a surprise to no one, sex also seems to increase overall happiness. In 2004, when economists analyzed data from 16,000 American adults including information on income, sexual activity, and happiness, they concluded that increasing the frequency of sex from once a month to once a week might increase happiness to the same extent as a $50,000 bonus.[8] In another survey, 1,000 employed women left no question as to where their priorities were when they rated sex as the activity that brought them the greatest happiness.[9]

So if enjoyment is your goal in life, it might be wise to spend less time arguing or worrying, and more time, you know, taking care of business.

But as with all the vices discussed in this book, moderation and pursuing sex in an enjoyable manner is the key. Forcing oneself to have more non-enjoyable, non-loving sex will *not* make you happier. Researchers at Carnegie Mellon University learned this when they recruited sixty-four adult couples and asked half of them to double their rate of sexual activity. Perhaps unsurprisingly, this prescription for more sex didn't lead to more enjoyment, and participants who were coaxed into more sex actually were less happy.[10]

As we've said again and again, the whole point of a good vice is doing something you enjoy in a manner that's enjoyable. Forcing yourself to do something you think you're *supposed* to think is fun is rarely fun.

When it comes to sex in popular culture, one topic that often doesn't get much attention is the evolutionary function of the act: making babies.

In regard to pregnancy, couples often fall into one of two camps, either trying very hard to get pregnant or trying very hard not to get pregnant.

Avoiding pregnancies has become a significant industry for pharmaceutical companies, and you can hardly get through a commercial break on TV now without seeing ads for intrauterine devices (IUDs), birth control pills, or other birth control methods. Many of these work by tricking a woman's body, which can have long-term adverse health effects.

While birth control methods are best decided on a couple-by-couple basis, those in a committed relationship should lean toward more natural, less invasive, and less potentially toxic methods.

On the flip side, for those who actually want to get pregnant, until recently so-called expert medical advice often was confusing and sometimes completely wrong. When couples have waited a long time to conceive, they may think they can just stop birth control and conceive overnight. In fact, there are only a few days a month when conception is likely. Sometimes it takes time, on occasion a lot of time and a lot of, well, sex. So be patient.

People often spend thousands of dollars on fertility clinics almost immediately after spending years trying to prevent pregnancy, but it often is best to first try eating right, exercising, lowering one's stress, and having lots of loving sex for quite a while.

Steak and sex, my favorite pair.
I have 'em both the same way—very rare.

—RODNEY DANGERFIELD

Lest our readers mistake our meaning in this chapter, we are not advocating careless promiscuity. There's ample evidence that committed relationships are the ones that offer the greatest rewards, and these extend well beyond the bedroom. As one New

York newspaper bluntly put it: "Being single will kill you faster than obesity, study says."[11,12]

A mammoth survey of 127,545 American adults found married men were healthier and generally lived longer than single, divorced, or widowed men. Some wondered if these results were skewed by healthy men's being more likely to marry, but the opposite actually is true: Unhealthy men are generally more likely to tie the knot. And the benefits of marriage seem to extend beyond just companionship. Those who live with others are generally healthier than those who live alone, and married men are even healthier—and also get a lifetime of invaluable driving advice.[13]

While sex is healthy, it's the quality, not the quantity, of "scoring" that counts. Yes, sex in and of itself can be healthy, but a loving relationship is far healthier. So find someone you care about and who cares about you and get your game on.

As the classic rock band Jefferson Airplane advises: "You better find somebody to love."

CHAPTER SIX

COFFEE

Hug a Mug

■ ■ ■

No one can understand the truth
until he drinks of coffee's frothy goodness.
—SHEIK ANSARI DJEZERI HANBALL ABD-AL-KADIR

IN BRIEF: The notion that coffee is unhealthy appears to be a myth. Moderate coffee drinking, up to three to five cups a day, can lower the chances of death from all causes, helps with a variety of specific ailments, and can increase quality of life. Try to sometimes stop using sugar and lots of cream in your coffee. Fresh-roasted, well-made coffee has rich flavors that cream and sugar may obscure.

A nomad named Kaldi was roaming the mountains of Ethiopia with his herd of goats, at a date and time lost to antiquity, when he made a discovery that would change the world forever: coffee.

Or rather, his goats did. According to legend, his goats began to munch on the bright red cherries growing on the mountainside. When they ate these cherries they became energetic and did something utterly un-goat-like—they began to dance. Those bright red cherries are the berries that now fuel the multibillion-dollar coffee industry.

Whether Kaldi's story is true or not, by around the tenth century BC, the mountain people of Ethiopia were eating these cherries for their stimulating effect. The process of extracting the cherry's immense flavors by drying, husking, and roasting the seeds to make a drink spread throughout the Arab world through Muslim Sufi mystics, who used coffee as an aid to concentrate as they chanted the name of God.

Today coffee is one of the world's most traded commodities, with millions of cups consumed each day in the United States. And although "coffee will stunt your growth" is a refrain we've all heard over and over again, there's about as much truth to it as there is flavor in most gas-station coffee. And that's just one of the many negative misconceptions surrounding this falsely convicted "guilty" pleasure. A series of studies from the 1970s and '80s tied the drink to higher rates of cancer and heart disease, but they failed to adjust for a participant's cigarette habit or other unhealthy lifestyle choices. Not only does new research show coffee does not affect your growth, it also suggests that *not* drinking coffee just might stunt your health.

Beyond any other food, beverage, or lifestyle choice featured in this book, coffee is probably the least deserving of its reputation as a vice. Despite the fact that it is frequently blacklisted as a drink you should avoid or at least limit, a slew of studies have reported that moderate coffee drinking—three to five cups a day—could increase cardiovascular health and lower the risk of stroke and developing Parkinson's disease, Alzheimer's, and type 2 diabetes, as well as reduce the chance of death from all causes. Coffee has been linked to so many health benefits that coffee lovers should be dancing with the joy of Kaldi's goats.

In a paper published by the American Heart Association in 2014, researchers conducted a systematic review of thirty-six studies with a combined sample size of more than 1,270,000 participants that looked at long-term consumption of coffee and its association with the risk of cardiovascular disease. These researchers found moderate coffee drinkers were at the lowest risk for problems.[1] Previous studies found similar results and suggested coffee also decreases the likelihood of a stroke.[2] Even excessive coffee guzzling (often defined as more than five cups a day) has been shown to have little or no adverse health side effects.[3]

Imagine if coffee were a new drug developed for a pharmaceutical company. Not only would it make billions, but also the advertising campaign associated with it might be big enough to move the Cialis and Viagra commercials out of prime time. After all, coffee has very few proven side effects and people love it.

So why does it have such a bad reputation?

The answer might be that coffee keeps some pretty unsavory company, most notably sugar. When we talk about the benefits of coffee, we can't stress enough that we're talking about straight black coffee, which generally has no calories, not the milk-shake-with-some-coffee-added beverages many people choose. Popular sugary coffee drinks at some major chains can have more than 400 calories. Even if we avoid the super-sugary drinks, coffee can pack something of a caloric wallop. An average-size coffee with cream and sugar has about 120 calories, while an average cappuccino has more than 100 calories.

In addition to its unhealthy stir-in ingredients, coffee often is paired with equally unhealthy practices and can serve as an enabler for bad habits like staying up too late or cramming for work or school. We turn to coffee to limit the effect of hangovers and to help us stay awake longer or get up earlier than we should.

The "magic" ingredient within coffee beans is caffeine, one of the world's most consumed drugs. Caffeine interferes with the way the chemical adenosine works in our bodies. In normal conditions, adenosine acts as a central nervous system depressant, promoting sleep and suppressing arousal by slowing down nerve activity. But when caffeine is absorbed into our blood, nerve cell adenosine receptors mistake caffeine for adenosine, binding to it instead of adenosine. This gives us that wonderful "coffee high" and helps fuel the beverage's benefits as a powerful antioxidant, a low-calorie natural brain stimulant, and a limiter of hyperglycemia. But if we abuse the drink, this delightful jolt of energy can backfire on us, causing anxiety and stress and temporarily raising blood pressure, all of which can be detrimental to our overall health.

All these negative secondary effects are easy to rectify. You can avoid sugar and high calories by drinking your coffee black. Few things on earth taste worse than poor-quality black coffee, but coffee aficionados often prefer black coffee because high-quality, consciously harvested Arabica coffee has rich, sweet flavors that are distinctly different depending on the region of the globe where the beans were grown. These flavors are almost entirely obscured by milk and sugar. All that being said, adding a little milk or cream still doesn't negate coffee's potential health benefits. For some people, adding a little cream to darker-roasted coffee can be a delightful treat. And a well-made cappuccino is truly a heavenly elixir.

You can also avoid making coffee a crutch for poor lifestyle choices by not treating it like a daily injection of energy. Although coffee is powered by the drug-like substance caffeine, it shouldn't be consumed like an injected stimulant to jolt you awake first thing in the morning; instead, make it a high-quality delicious ritual that you enjoy and look forward to experiencing. Think of coffee's ancient history and steep your drinking of the beverage in ritual. Coffeehouses have traditionally been spots where artists and scientists would meet to exchange ideas, and you should use the jolt of energy the drink affords to stimulate your intellect and creative side, not just to get through the day and manage stress. Take a few minutes with a newspaper or a good book with your morning coffee, or meet up with a friend or coworker.

In addition to coffee, black, white, and green teas have many well-known and accepted health benefits, and we and our patients drink tea often. We haven't devoted a chapter to it because, well, other than at the Boston Tea Party, tea isn't really considered a vice. Besides, since the American Revolution, coffee has been the American drink of choice. After all, it was coffee, not tea, that the settlers often took instead of more food on their wagon trains for the perilous journey west. Still, as mentioned, tea can be a very healthy drink. The average cup contains about a third of the caffeine of coffee and its methylxanthine theophylline has been used for decades as a bronchodilator and a treatment for asthma. So vice or not, go ahead and enjoy tea along with or instead of coffee.

Potentially more troubling to the health conscious are the coffee-like stains on the reputation of the beverage itself. But, as mentioned earlier, those studies from the 1970s and '80s associating the drink with higher rates of cancer and heart disease had significant issues with their methodology, and those results have not been reproduced in decades. In fact, more recent, larger studies have suggested the opposite is true. One study saw a link between coffee and an overall decrease in cancer,[4] and several recent meta-studies have found that drinking coffee was associated with a significantly reduced chance of death from all causes.[5]

In addition, some studies are equivocal if not downright perplexing. Data collected from the Singapore Chinese Health Study, which is a population-based prospective cohort that recruited 63,257 Chinese participants, age forty-five to seventy-four, who resided in Singapore from 1993 to 1998, found that "participants who drank less than 1 cup of coffee per week or more than 2 cups of coffee per day had a significant reduction in risk of hypertension compared to those who drank 1 cup per day." Therefore, according to this study, someone with mild hypertension who drinks one cup of coffee a day might be better off either discontinuing most coffee or drinking a lot more.[6]

In 2016, a prestigious panel of twenty-three scientists convened by the International Agency for Research on Cancer (IARC), an agency of the World Health Organization (WHO), "found no conclusive evidence for a carcinogenic effect of drinking coffee," though they noted drinking extremely hot beverages of any kind "probably causes cancer of the esophagus in humans." The decision was a rare reversal by the panel, which had declared coffee a likely carcinogen in 1991. The new conclusions were reached after scientists on the panel reviewed more than one thousand studies on coffee.[7]

That all being said, drinking coffee on an empty stomach,

particularly strong black coffee or even coffee with only a little bit of milk or cream, can sometimes precipitate digestive issues, and for some people it may be better to drink coffee a little later in the day. There also can be physical withdrawal symptoms, including severe headaches, when regular coffee drinkers abruptly stop drinking coffee.

Taken all together, the research is in coffee's favor, suggesting it is a mostly harmless and potentially healthy drink. Not only will it not stunt your growth, coffee for adults in sugar-free moderation is an enjoyable practice with great health potential. We're not likely to see commercials touting the health benefits of this wonderful "drug," but it might be a good idea to talk to your doctor and see if coffee is right for you. The research suggests it probably is.

CHAPTER SEVEN

CHOCOLATE

Love Without Words

■ ■ ■

All you need is love. But a little chocolate now and then
doesn't hurt.

—CHARLES M. SCHULZ

IN BRIEF: A little chocolate can go a long way to sweeten up your life
and may even be healthy. Chocolate has been shown in various studies to lower the risk of heart disease and strokes and possibly to slow
the rate of cognitive decline.

The Aztecs believed chocolate was a gift from Quetzalcoatl, the
god of wisdom. This delicious food comes from the seeds of cacao
trees, which produce the cocoa "beans" (which, like coffee, are
actually seeds). These were first used in fermented beverages in
Mesoamerica several thousand years ago.

This gift from the gods was appreciated by sixteenth-century
European colonizers, who found that when mixed with sugar,
chocolate became even more heavenly. Sugar-infused chocolate
became a part of European culture, and although the chocolate
trade proved a financial boon, it came with a cost. As Europeans
began to consume unhealthy amounts of chocolate and sugar,

their teeth began to rot and their health deteriorated. Chocolate's reputation was ultimately stained. It, like too many treats in our culture, became a guilty pleasure, with sometimes too great an emphasis on the "guilty" part of the equation.

Fortunately, there has been growing awareness more recently that when it comes to health, chocolate really might be a gift from the gods. For a study published in the journal *Heart* in 2015, researchers did a meta-analysis with a combined sample size of more than 150,000 people. They found that regular consumers of chocolate had a 21 percent lower risk of stroke, a 29 percent lower risk of developing heart disease, and a whopping 45 percent lower risk of dying of heart disease (though not all 150,000 people were studied for each of these conditions). Participants eating up to 3.5 ounces of chocolate a day enjoyed these benefits.

Unlike most studies in which the benefits were primarily associated with dark chocolate, in this meta-analysis many participants did not regularly eat dark chocolate. While researchers cautioned that they couldn't conclude that chocolate was the only reason for these benefits, they said, "There does not appear to be any evidence to say that chocolate should be avoided in those who are concerned about cardiovascular risk."[1]

These results are not unusual. In 2016, researchers in Sweden did a prospective study of 67,640 men and women and found, as previous researchers have, that chocolate consumption is associated with a lower risk of heart disease.[2] A 2010 German study of 19,357 people found regular moderate chocolate consumption appeared to lower the risk of heart disease, in part by reducing blood pressure.[3] And a decreased chance of heart disease is just the beginning of the potential health effects of moderate chocolate consumption.

Many years ago, we would tell people to stop eating sugar, including most chocolate. Back then we believed, as most medical professionals did at the time, that chocolate was inherently unhealthy. Then we noticed that French patients who continued to enjoy chocolate as part of their afternoon ritual weighed less and often had better blood work than many U.S. patients. We learned that like wine, chocolate is a part of life in French culture and might be at least partially responsible for the French Paradox.

As time went on, there were more and more healthy patients who enjoyed dark chocolate in moderation. We, and the authors of several new studies, hypothesized it might provide a health benefit for those who consumed small amounts of it.

In addition to lowering the risk of heart disease, eating small amounts of chocolate has been linked to a lower risk of strokes, lower blood pressure, and a slower rate of cognitive decline and possibly the onset of Alzheimer's.

In fact, if you forget to eat chocolate, you *might* just start forgetting a whole bunch of other things. In a study published in the *Journal of Alzheimer's Disease* in 2016, researchers in Portugal found that chocolate eaters had about a 40 percent lower risk of cognitive decline in a group of about five hundred participants age sixty-five years and older.[4]

Researchers at Columbia University Irving Medical Center took things a step further. In a 2014 study they recruited thirty-seven healthy adults age fifty to sixty-eight. Participants who drank a mixture made specifically for the experiment that was high in cocoa flavanols performed better on memory tests than those who drank a low-flavanol mixture. Although the sample size was small and the mixture was made specifically for the study, the results suggested greater potential for cocoa's memory-boosting abilities. Participants drank the mixture for only three months and performed like people several decades younger on the study's memory test, roughly 25 percent better than those who drank the non-cocoa mixture.[5]

So what is it that makes this tasty treat healthy?

Chocolate, particularly dark chocolate, is extremely rich in antioxidants like polyphenols and flavonols. One study found that cocoa powder contains higher levels of antioxidants than many so-called super fruits, including blueberries, cranberries, and pomegranates.[6] Chocolate, like coffee, is a rich source of methylxanthines—these include theobromine in chocolate, theophylline in tea, and caffeine in coffee, all of which stimulate our bodies in slightly different ways. Even though chocolate contains theobromine, which is similar to caffeine, it does not seem to give the same "jolt" as coffee, but it does offer a sense of well-being to many.

There is some indication that humans have long sought out food and beverages containing methylxanthines at least in part because of the way they make us feel. In 2013, researchers argued in the journal *Nutrients* that the reason humans have historically been drawn to chocolate and are still attracted to it is its positive influence on our mental state.

It is likely that humans have stuck to any brew containing compounds with psychoactive properties, resulting in a better daily life, i.e., more efficient thinking, exploring, hunting, etc. . . . Historical and anthropological data demonstrate that man has searched for nutrients and/or beverages that contained substances that helped not only calorically, but also in terms of well-being.

The study's authors concluded that chocolate is particularly good for that sense of well-being because theobromine is more active in it than caffeine and does not generally produce anxiety or insomnia.[7]

These positive properties are found in greater abundance in dark chocolate than in milk chocolate, which has fewer antioxidants and less actual cocoa. White chocolate has even fewer antioxidants and less cocoa; in fact, it is not even really chocolate, though it does contain cocoa flavorings. We recommend eating dark chocolate that is at least 70 percent chocolate or higher. There are a greater number of studies supporting dark chocolate's health benefits, and it has less sugar and fat than milk chocolate.

Keep chocolate in your diet only if you don't have issues with the metabolism of sugar, because most chocolate (other than pure cocoa) does contain sugar, and as with the other vices discussed in this book, only if it's something you already enjoy. Before you empty your vegetable drawer and replace the food in your cabinets with chocolate, remember that fruits and vegetables are still healthier than chocolate. Most research suggesting chocolate's health benefits have focused on dark chocolate consumption; and when we talk about chocolate, we are primarily talking about high-quality dark chocolate, not the junk-food, ultra-industrialized varieties you'll find in most grocery store aisles, which are the true monsters of the Halloween season. Chocolate can be unhealthy when abused because it can contain lots of sugar and calories. Those who totally give in to their sweet-tooth demons ultimately can suffer from conditions like type 2 diabetes, and a diet too high in sugar has been linked to an increased risk of Alzheimer's and stroke.

But to those who eat chocolate while employing that magic word *moderation,* there is possibly much to be gained, and we believe those who eat chocolate are not only getting beneficial antioxidants and some of the health benefits from the treat itself, but are also getting the joy of eating something they love.

It should be noted that there may be a positive bias when studies are funded by industry, as many medical studies, including chocolate studies, are. We therefore advise using common sense and prudence, and we don't suggest eating gobs of chocolate instead of fresh fruits and vegetables.

Don't snack on a bowl of bonbons all day, or chow down on gas-station candy on your stressful commute to work. Like other "good vices" in this book, it's best to turn chocolate eating into something you look forward to and relish. Enjoy it with your afternoon tea or coffee, or as a small dessert after dinner. Go for quality over quantity by indulging in handcrafted or single-origin chocolate if you can find it. Remember, savor and enjoy each bite. Focus on the richness of the flavors, the hints of tropical fruit that can be detected on the tongue, and the smoothness of good chocolate. If you do, the health returns from chocolate will likely be, in a word, sweet.

CHAPTER EIGHT

SWEET-TOOTH BONANZA

Honey, Maple Syrup, and Sugarcane

■ ■ ■

The most important thing to remember about
food labels is that you should avoid foods
that have labels.

—JOEL FURHMAN

IN BRIEF: Honey and maple syrup have a host of health benefits when consumed in moderation, as do berries and fruit that contain natural sugars. Processed sugar is not good for us, but is okay once in a while as a treat. Avoid high-fructose corn syrup and artificial sweeteners found in diet sodas.

Their daughter would be raised without sugar. That's what Harry and Patty decided when they had their first child in the early 1980s. Harry recently had graduated from the National University of Natural Medicine in Portland, Oregon; Patty was a nurse and soon to be a nurse practitioner; and the couple was, to put it mildly, health-conscious.

Instead of candy, chocolate, ice cream, or any sugar-powered sweets, their daughter Ilana had fresh fruit as a treat. They thought by having her avoid all but natural sugar early on, she would be healthier in the short term and less likely to develop a sweet tooth in the long term.

The plan didn't exactly work.

When Ilana was about four, a family friend brought a box of cookies for an after-dinner treat because he knew the Ofgang house would be dessert-free. Though Ilana had had very limited exposure to sugar, the contents of that box called to her as strongly as the song of the Sirens lured Odysseus.

At the start of dinner that evening no one could find her. When her parents called her name, they got no response. Then they heard mouse-like scurrying coming from inside the pantry in which they had hidden the round box of delectable cookies. Opening the door, they found Ilana with her head in the box gorging on the sweet treats, oblivious to the outside world, experiencing something close to sugar-induced nirvana.

The incident demonstrated that when it came to sugar and their daughter, abstinence didn't seem to work. Despite their best efforts, their sweet little daughter had an innate sweet tooth.

She is not unique in this. Regardless of their background, religion, or ethnicity, many humans share a common trait: They were born craving sweetness.

Darwinian evolution through the ages taught our ancestors to seek out sugar—the greatest natural food on earth for human babies, breast milk, is naturally sweet. Sugar was relatively rare for most of human history and was an important form of energy in food, but excess sugars in our bloodstream are converted by the liver to glycogen and fatty acids. Sugar's fat-producing abilities may have been beneficial in the hunter-gatherer era, as humans needed to store large amounts of fat to survive during periods when food was scarce.

With the development of large-scale agriculture and the rise of civilizations, starch became much more abundant. Moses led the Israelites out of slavery in Egypt and promised to take them to a land flowing with milk and honey, as the latter was the sweetest food regularly available in ancient days. Back then the ratio of sugar consumption to energy burning was still relatively good. Our collective sugar craving didn't become a problem until pure sugar became readily available with the planting of large sugar plantations in the New World. Unfortunately, humans' demand for sugar did not wane as the supply increased.

That led to the present day, when we have grocery aisles full of sugary products—from candy and cakes to soda, orange juice, and many other purportedly healthy beverages. Our deep-rooted instincts urge us to reach for those cakes, slurp those sodas, and gobble up those candies. Many have compared our sugar craving to an addict's craving for drugs, and indeed sugar, like addictive drugs, releases dopamine in our brain, causing intense pleasure and cravings to repeat the experience.

Fortunately, we've got some good news.

In this chapter, we're here to talk about how to work with rather than against those instincts by consuming small amounts of sweet and healthy products such as fruits and berries, honey and maple syrup, as well as moderate amounts of real sugar (preferably direct from the actual sugarcane), not those chemical-ridden unhealthy substitutes. This will turn our sweet tooth into a sweet component of our health, rather than something we're always fighting.

During late winter and early spring, our family would often tap the maple trees outside our home. A New England tradition, the harvesting of sap from the maple tree was developed by indigenous tribes in the Americas who realized that when concentrated, this sap created a sweet, delicious syrup.

To get the best maple syrup, you must boil the sap a long time, waiting until it turns a dark golden color and has a syrupy consistency. Boil it too long and it hardens into maple candy or evaporates entirely.

Making healthy and delicious maple syrup, though, is not without peril. There were times when we didn't get the timing right and it was too watery. One time we forgot to check on the sap and boiled it for far too long. The liquid evaporated, the bottom of the pot began to burn on the outdoor grill, and it charred the deck where we were making the syrup. Luckily, we caught it before it started a bigger fire.

Despite the difficulties involved, making maple syrup was well worth the effort. The syrup we managed to make successfully was rich, sweet, and better than any we'd ever tasted that had been commercially produced. It also was healthy.

Real maple syrup—not that sugary, watery, synthetic fraud served atop pancakes at way too many restaurants and diners—has a lower glycemic index, a value assigned based on how quickly foods cause increases in blood sugar, than cane sugar. Maple syrup's glycemic index is about 54, while cane sugar's glycemic index is about 65.

In addition, maple syrup is rich in antioxidants and may pack the same health wallop as berries, red wine, green tea, flax, whole grains, and other healthy foods. In 2011, researchers led by Dr. Navindra Seeram at the University of Rhode Island found in the laboratory setting that maple syrup had many more healthy compounds than previously thought and that polyphenols in maple syrup might inhibit enzymes that are involved in the conversion of carbohydrates to sugar, and as such, might help in fighting type 2 diabetes.[1]

Additional research conducted by Seeram suggests maple syrup also may be helpful in creating a healthy gut with the proper balance of good bacteria, which can protect against irritable bowel syndrome and chronic inflammation, both of which may be associated with a host of diseases such as dementia. In addition, maple syrup may have qualities similar to those in red wine when it comes to protecting brain health and reducing the chances of cognitive decline.[2]

Maple syrup is rich in vitamins including zinc, manganese, potassium, and calcium. Zinc helps keep the body's white blood cell count high, while manganese helps with fat and carbohydrate metabolism, calcium absorption, and blood sugar regulation along with other brain and nerve functions.

Much like the old adage that says wood heats twice, once when you labor to cut it and again when you burn it in a woodstove, making your own maple syrup rewards you twice—first when you are out among the beautiful maple trees in the fresh, brisk winter air gathering the maple sap, and later when you savor the delicious treat on top of pancakes made from freshly ground whole grains.

Maple syrup isn't the only healthy sweetener. Honey has been favorably linked to everything from weight loss to allergy relief, and it has antibacterial properties. Like maple syrup, honey is rich in antioxidants, with high concentrations of polyphenols, which may have a role in preventing degenerative diseases, especially cardiovascular disorders and cancer. Researchers at San Diego State University found that consuming honey instead of sugar lowered blood sugar and reduced weight gain in rats.[3] Another study found raw honey could activate hormones that suppress the appetites of women.[4]

Participants in a 2013 study who ate high doses of honey (one gram per kilogram of body weight daily) for eight weeks decreased their allergy symptoms.[5] Some advocate local unfiltered raw honey as particularly effective in fighting allergies, and patients have shared many anecdotes about a decrease in allergy symptoms from eating local honey.

On top of these benefits, this natural substance is a powerful bacteria fighter and has been used since ancient times to dress wounds. Recent studies have shown that this old treatment is effective, sometimes even against drug-resistant bacteria.[6,7]

So honey and maple are good, but what about sugar?

A little sugar from natural sources is fine for most people. Fruit is sweet because of the natural sugars in it. This sugar is not bad for you if you have a few fruits a day and aren't diabetic. But what about having real honest-to-goodness sugar? You know, the kind you find in ice cream, not apples? This is best to consume only in moderation, and where possible, as raw pressed sugarcane.

Avoid high-fructose corn syrup—a corn-based sweetener that

has seen ever-increasing use in industrialized food since the 1970s—and stick to traditional sugar made from pure sugarcane. Or better yet, head down to your local ethnic market and get an actual whole cane.

Consuming large amounts of both high-fructose corn syrup and refined sugar is very unhealthy and can cause increased weight gain and all that comes with it—including the increased chance of diabetes and heart disease. And as we noted earlier, a diet too high in sugar could be linked to an increased risk of Alzheimer's and stroke. But avoiding sugar completely and trying to replace it with other unnatural sweeteners can be bad as well. Drinking diet sodas, which use artificial sweeteners instead of sugar, is not a good trade-off.

Sharon P. Fowler, a researcher in the Department of Medicine at the University of Texas Health Science Center at San Antonio, has found links between diet soda consumption and weight gain in multiple studies. In 2008, she looked at 3,682 adults and found that diet soda drinkers were more likely to gain weight.[8] In 2015, she studied 749 adults age sixty-five and older, finding that occasional and regular diet soda drinkers gained nearly three times as much as those who did not drink diet soda when factors such as exercise and smoking were ruled out.[9] These findings have been disputed by the soft drink industry, but they jibe perfectly with what we've noticed from patients who are diet soda drinkers. We see no great harm in an occasional diet or regular soda. Seltzer or mineral water with a squeeze of lemon or lime might be a better alternative. Believe it or not, another alternative is fresh, natural tap water. Cold tap water with a splash of lime or lemon can be more enjoyable and refreshing than you might think.

One more tidbit that's so sweet we had trouble believing it. According to a diet featured in *Prevention* magazine, "You can lose weight and eat ice cream once a day, too. The trick is moderation, and eating healthy meals the rest of the day. While on the diet, women may have 1 cup of ice cream, and men may have 1½ cups per day."[10]

Even if, like us, you're too skeptical to eat ice cream every day, as we learned earlier, total abstinence can be too hard and sometimes unrealistic. So try to use things like honey, maple syrup, or whole sugarcane whenever possible, or failing that, use real unadulterated sugar instead of artificial sweeteners. Be honest with yourself and acknowledge that the vast majority of us are going to have sugar from time to time, so most of us are best off trying to limit, not eliminate, our consumption.

Rather than fighting our sweet-tooth cravings with total abstinence, we can give in to them with honey and maple syrup and, every once in a while, just a little bit of real, delicious, energy-providing sugar.

CHAPTER NINE

BE FREE OF FAT-FREE

■ ■ ■

What the Soviet Union was to the ideology of
Marxism, the Low-Fat Campaign is to the ideology
of nutritionism—its supreme test and,
as now is coming clear, its most abject failure.
—MICHAEL POLLAN, *IN DEFENSE OF FOOD*

IN BRIEF: Low-fat diets have been debunked as ineffective from a weight loss and health perspective. Studies show natural, full-fat dairy, eggs, olive oil, nuts, and other fat-rich foods are healthy when consumed in moderation.

In the 1960s, the war on fat began. Early in that tumultuous decade, the American Heart Association started recommending a diet low in saturated fat and cholesterol from animal products. As America's actual war in Vietnam intensified and the hippie counterculture grew, changing American society forever, a dramatic cultural shift occurred at dinner, lunch, and breakfast tables across the country.

Fat became Public Health Enemy No. 1. Fatty but healthy foods—provisions that came from the earth, were full of vitamins and other nutrients, and were free of impossible-to-pronounce ingredients—got pushed off grocery store shelves and out of the diets of the health-conscious.

Creamy whole milk, already adulterated by pasteurization and homogenization, was replaced with that thin, flavorless impostor known as skim milk; full-fat yogurt, rich in probiotics and good bacteria, was nearly hunted into extinction; and eating eggs, especially the yolks, became cause for an "egg-xistential" crisis.

From the beginning flavor was an acknowledged casualty of the war, but the public was told it was a necessary sacrifice for better health. Avoiding fat, generations of people were taught, would decrease weight, lower blood pressure, and reduce the chance of heart disease, among other benefits. None of these claims have withstood the test of scientific scrutiny, and most of the reasons behind the start of the war on fat have proved to be as bogus as the reasons for many actual wars.

"It is now increasingly recognized that the low-fat campaign has been based on little scientific evidence and may have caused unintended health consequences," wrote a group of prominent nutrition scientists at the Harvard T. H. Chan School of Public Health way back in 2001. The paper noted that while "in the public's mind, the words 'dietary fat' have become synonymous with obesity and heart disease, whereas the words 'low-fat' and 'fat-free' have been synonymous with 'heart health,' few studies found an association between low-fat diets and decreased incidence of heart disease, while many have failed to find an association." Furthermore, "There was little or no association between high cholesterol diets and heart disease and little direct evidence linking higher egg consumption and increased risk of CHD [coronary heart disease]."[1]

These conclusions have been expanded on since, and there is a growing—most likely on a misguided fat-free diet—body of evidence that the low-fat diet is not, as we've long been told, a healthy one. A 2017 study in *The Lancet*, one of medicine's most prestigious journals, looked at 135,335 people age thirty-five to seventy from eighteen countries. The results suggested that knocking out the fat, as the boxer-turned-grill-promoter George Foreman once advised, is not all it's cracked up to be. Instead, the study found there was a significantly reduced risk of death for those who ate more fat. Andrew Mente, an epidemiologist at McMaster University in Ontario and one of the authors of the study, told *The New York Times* that current fat "guidelines recommend low saturated fat, and some recommend really low amounts. Our study, which captures intake at the lowest levels, shows that this may be harmful."[2]

Those who ate the highest percentage of carbohydrates had a 28 percent increased risk of death compared to those who ate the lowest percentage of carbs. At the same time, folks with the highest fat intake, who on average consumed 35.3 percent of their daily calories from fat, had a 23 percent reduced risk of death compared with those with the lowest percent of calories from fat (an average of 10.6 percent of calories from fat).[3]

The Harvard T. H. Chan School of Public Health currently advises: "Contrary to past dietary advice promoting low-fat diets, newer research shows that healthy fats are necessary and beneficial for health," and modern studies show "no link between the overall percentage of calories from fat and any important health outcome, including cancer, heart disease, and weight gain."[4]

We've noticed over the years that those who followed a more

natural, primal-like diet—one rich in fermented probiotic foods and inspected raw butter, milk, cheese, and eggs, from pasture-raised and pasture-finished animals—aged gracefully and were for the most part not overweight. The upshot is that unless a doctor specifically prescribes a low-fat diet, studies indicate that it is reasonable to judiciously indulge in previously shunned foods like whole (raw) milk, whole yogurt, and eggs from free-roaming chickens, and in general to stop fat-shaming what you eat.

Today the war on dietary fat is rumored to be over, but you wouldn't know it while exploring a modern grocery store or reading the recommendations from many diet books.

During a recent trip to the grocery store, we had a hard time finding regular full-fat yogurt, though we easily found plenty of nonfat products, including nonfat cookies, muffins, milk, cheese, butter, and cream. There were other odd nonfat substitutes, and even substitutes of substitutes—vegetarian turkey burgers, anyone? (We're not exactly sure how a vegetarian mix nails the flavor of a turkey burger trying to taste like a beef burger.)

Particularly ironic is how little all these fat-free products have done to produce, you know, weight loss. Since the 1960s, when low-fat diets became all the rage, the average American man ballooned from about 166 pounds to 195 pounds, while the average American woman weighed in at around 140 in the 1960s, but by 2010, was tipping the scale at about 166 pounds.[5]

Men and women have grown a bit taller on average, which accounts for some but certainly not all of the weight gain. A more likely culprit is our obsession with fat-free products, as over the same time period, the percentage of fat in our diets declined from 45 percent to 33 percent.[6]

And the rising numbers on our scales aren't the only evidence against a fat-free diet. A 2016 study in *The American Journal of Clinical Nutrition* studied 18,438 women and found those who consumed the most high-fat dairy products lowered their risk of being overweight or obese by 8 percent.[7]

The reasons for these results are unclear; it's possible that since fat is very filling, when people cut it from their diets, they replace it with sugar or carbohydrates. Either way, the *weight* of the evidence against fat-free diets is almost as overwhelming as our actual weight.

This doesn't mean you should ignore every fat-avoiding instinct you have and start gorging on giant milk shakes and burgers slathered in mayonnaise. (Several of the very high-fat diet fads touted on social media, especially when not followed to the letter, can easily lead to increased weight gain and illness.) But it does mean you can stop scouring the grocery store for fat-free labels and start drinking whole milk and eating yogurt. And according to recent studies, you also can start eating eggs again, including the yolks.

Fat is a necessary nutrient. It helps us absorb fat-soluble vitamins like A, D, E, and K. Vitamin D is important for healthy bones, cardiac health, and the immune system. Low levels of vitamin D correlate with the symptoms of IBD (inflammatory bowel disease like colitis and Crohn's). Vitamin A is important for good vision, healthy bone growth, skin health, and reproduction. It also helps the immune system. Similarly, vitamin E helps ensure good vision, healthy bone growth, and reproduction. Vitamin K not only plays an important part in blood clotting, but helps prevent heart disease and supports bone growth as well. So, you see, fat is not just a guilty indulgence but an important part of a healthy diet.

Full-fat dairy products, especially inspected and certified raw dairy, also are a source of calcium and protein. While skim milk advertises the same nutrients and fewer calories than whole milk, evidence shows that whole milk drinkers are healthier than nonfat milk drinkers, and full-fat dairy eaters in general are healthier than low-fat dairy consumers. One study of 3,333 adults found that people who had high levels of by-products of full-fat dairy in their blood had a 46 percent lower risk of getting diabetes.[8]

Additionally, raw milk—milk that has not been pasteurized (boiled)—has more nutrients, protective enzymes and probiotics, or good bacteria. Raw milk was shown to reduce the instances of asthma and allergies in a study of more than 8,000 children in Germany, Austria, and Switzerland.[9] Researchers found similar results in Amish children living in Indiana.[10]

Our family almost exclusively drank raw milk that was milked by hand by "Farmer Ed" on the dairy farm just down the road from our hilltop log house. The rich, delicious natural dairy helped keep us healthy and happy even during the long, cold New England winters we endured.

When it comes to cheese, making it low in fat often robs it of many of its healthiest components; and raw milk cheese, sometimes imported from other countries, is especially healthy.

Whole (full-fat) yogurt is a particularly important source of probiotics, with its live strains of good bacteria that can help boost the immune system and support a healthy gut.

What about that delicious egg we couldn't eat for years? It

turns out that the cholesterol in eggs is not associated with high blood cholesterol levels or heart disease, and the yolk of the egg is an excellent source of those important fat-soluble vitamins. This is especially true when the eggs come from free-range chickens.

Even the government of Ireland has thrown considerable weight behind the promotion of delicious, creamy butter from pasture-fed cows, which fortunately is available now in supermarkets around the world.

Beyond the dairy aisle, there are a number of healthy and—yes—fatty products you should seek out the next time you shop. Omega-3 fatty acids, a type of fat found in fish, nuts, and seeds, are a health boon. They can help lower elevated blood fat (triglycerides), decrease stiffness and joint pain from arthritis, possibly lower levels of depression, help visual and neurological development in infants, help stave off the onset of Alzheimer's, and increase lung function for people suffering from asthma. Omega-3 fatty acids are naturally found in tasty foods like fish, especially sardines, wild salmon (which has higher levels than farmed), and anchovies, as well as nuts and seeds, with particularly high levels in walnuts.

Areas of Italy where people live the longest tend to be where people walk outside often; have close, ongoing family and social relationships; and consume fresh herbs like rosemary as well as fish and lots of anchovies. Although nuts are high in calories and therefore often avoided in our fat-fearing culture, they are a wonderful source of nutrition and roughage, and there is a good deal of research suggesting they can improve heart health and reduce the risk of death from heart disease and other causes.

The extra-large benefits of various fatty foods abound. Fresh-pressed extra-virgin olive oil is an important part of the Mediterranean diet consumed by some of the world's healthiest and longest-living individuals. Avocados, though high in fat, are brimming with nearly twenty vitamins and minerals that, among other things, help us maintain good cholesterol levels. They also are great for vision. Coconuts and coconut oil not only provide a beneficial fat that is delicious to ingest but have been used for years by indigenous people to help beautify and nourish their hair and skin.

The low-fat frenzy has encouraged us to eat only white meat and lean meat, but that leaves out a lot of healthy parts of the animal. Most cultures eat chicken and turkey gizzards and products such as the liver, but in the United States people often avoid these vitamin-rich organ foods. Liver and other organ meats contain large amounts of protein and easy-to-absorb iron, as well as a host of vitamins, including all the B vitamins. These types of foods can often be found at ethnic supermarkets. After selecting a full range of fruits and vegetables at one of these stores, add some organ meat to the cart if you already eat meat occasionally.

Wait a minute! inquisitive readers might be thinking at this point. *If fat-free diets have been debunked and fat is healthy, why hasn't the health community done a better job of sharing the news with us? Why haven't grocery stores and many dietitians caught up?*

The answer is . . . we're not sure.

In his well-known book *In Defense of Food*, Michael Pollan addresses the same question. He writes: "No one in charge—not in the government, not in the public health community—has dared to come out and announce: *Um, you know everything we've been telling you for the last thirty years about the links between dietary fat and heart disease? And fat and cancer? And fat and fat? Well, this just in: It now appears that none of it was true. We sincerely regret the error.*"[11]

It's possible the fat-free industry has become such a big part of the food world that there's not enough monetary incentive to change. Some believe that fat-free products result in lower costs for food producers, since the fat taken from *your* milk, yogurt, and cheese then can be used in other products.

If that's true, it's not surprising, as economics helped get us here.

The original vilifying of fat may *not* have been an honest mistake by the medical community, but perhaps a profit-driven muddying of the waters. In 2016, a paper in *JAMA Internal Medicine* revealed how the sugar industry paid scientists in the 1960s to downplay the link between sugar and heart disease and to promote fat as the villain instead. The research detailed how the Sugar Research Foundation, a sugar industry group known today as the Sugar Association, paid three Harvard scientists about $50,000 in today's dollars to publish a 1967 review of research on sugar and fat and their relationship to heart disease. The influential paper was published in *The New England Journal of Medicine*; it let sugar off the hook in regard to heart health, instead casting fat as the villain. "Our findings suggest the industry sponsored a research program in the 1960s and 1970s that successfully cast doubt about the hazards of sucrose while promoting fat as the dietary culprit in CHD [coronary heart disease]," state authors Cristin Kearns, Laura Schmidt, and Stanton Glantz.[12]

In 1954, the president of the Sugar Research Foundation gave a speech in which he said that if Americans could be persuaded to eat a diet lower in fat for health, they would need to replace that fat with something, and America's per capita sugar consumption could increase by a third.

In the 1960s, when reports began appearing that suggested sugar was a less desirable dietary source of calories than other carbohydrates, John Hickson, vice president and director of research for the foundation, recommended that the industry fund its own studies: "Then we can publish the data and refute our detractors."

By the mid-1960s, Hickson had enlisted the aforementioned Harvard scientists, including nutritionist D. Mark Hegsted (who went on to become the head of nutrition at the U.S. Department of Agriculture and in 1977 helped draft a forerunner to the federal government's dietary guidelines) and Dr. Fredrick J. Stare, chairman of Harvard's nutrition department. Hickson discussed the research with the scientists and viewed drafts. When the report was finished, he made it known he was happy with the results. "Let me assure you this is quite what we had in mind," he wrote to one of the scientists. Appearing in an influential journal, the paper had a significant impact that still is being felt today.

Before jumping full tilt into the full-fat counterrevolution, remember vices, including fat, are best enjoyed in moderation. Exercising and eating a mostly plant-based diet—one centered on fruits, vegetables, nuts, seeds, and berries—is best for most people. If you do eat meat, we suggest moderation and seeking out local pasture-raised and -finished meat.

In addition, be cautious about nutrition plans that praise high-fat diets at the expense of all other foods. Health and nutrition experts often are like passengers on an overcrowded boat. When everyone is on one side and they realize water is starting to pour onboard, they rush to the other side, only to have—you guessed it—the same problem.

Today many so-called experts are rushing away from the fat-free side of the boat toward the high-fat, low-carb, less-miraculous-than-advertised side. Because of this trend, fat is being replaced by a new villain of healthy eating, often considered as evil as Satan himself. The much-maligned topic of our next chapter is a food that actually is healthy for the vast majority of us, but you wouldn't know that anymore. In fact, in mixed company you might not even want to say its name out loud. We're only whispering it now: *bread.*

CHAPTER TEN

BREAKING BREAD MYTHS

■ ■ ■

*There is not a thing that is more positive
than bread.*
—FYODOR DOSTOEVSKY

IN BRIEF: Giving up all whole-grain bread is not healthier for everyone. For those who are not truly gluten intolerant or significantly allergic, eating whole grains regularly seems to improve heart health
and decrease the chance of death from all causes.

Referring to bread as a vice would have seemed absurd twenty
years ago. Historically, wars were fought over bread, revolutions
were started because of its shortage, and breaking bread became
a symbol not only of friendship but of peace and understanding.
Today, bread—that most basic and beloved of all modern human
foods, the very same substance your parents packed in your school
lunch box—has become perhaps the most hated food group in the
United States.

The reason for bread's fall from grace can be traced to one
single, apparently cursed word: *gluten*. One of the most consumed
proteins on the planet, gluten is formed by glutenin and gliadin

molecules coming together and creating a bond that when kneaded into dough results in a stretchy membrane, giving bread its chewy texture. It has replaced fat as the dietary bogeyman of our time and is blamed for everything from weight gain to allergies to irritable bowel syndrome (IBS) and long lines at airports. (Okay, so that last one is an exaggeration.)

For the small number of people who have celiac disease (less than 1 percent of the population), or some other severe gluten intolerance or allergy, gluten is indeed a dangerous substance to be avoided. But many of us should be more gluten tolerant. Some of the side effects of gluten have been exaggerated, and real bread, gluten and all, consumed in moderation actually is really good for the majority of us.

Bread made from freshly ground whole grains is filling and provides nutrients like vitamins E and B and minerals like iron, magnesium, selenium, and others. It is also a very rich source of dietary fiber, which can lower people's bad cholesterol or LDL, improving their heart health in the process.

A 2017 Harvard Medical School study looking at 64,714 women and 45,303 men found that those who consumed the lowest levels of gluten were 15 percent more likely to develop heart disease. This "heartening" study for bread eaters concluded, "The avoidance of gluten may result in reduced consumption of beneficial whole grains, which may affect cardiovascular risk. The promotion of gluten-free diets among people without celiac disease should not be encouraged."

And that's not all. Study authors noted these findings were particularly troubling because the number of people unnecessarily avoiding gluten seems to be on the rise. From 2009 to 2010, only

0.52 percent of the population who did not suffer from celiac disease had gluten-free diets, but by 2013–2014, that number had more than tripled to 1.69 percent of the celiac-free population.[1]

This is far from the only research singing bread's praises. For a 2016 report in *BMJ* (formerly the *British Medical Journal*), researchers looked at forty-five previous studies and concluded that compared with those who ate no wheat, those who consumed 90 grams of whole grains a day reduced their risk for all-cause mortality by 17 percent. They also provided further evidence that "whole grain intake is associated with a reduced risk of coronary heart disease, cardiovascular disease, and total cancer, and mortality from all causes, respiratory diseases, infectious diseases, diabetes, and all non-cardiovascular, non-cancer causes." Their conclusion was that such "findings support dietary guidelines that recommend increased intake of whole grain to reduce the risk of chronic diseases and premature mortality."[2]

Another 2016 analysis looked at fourteen prospective studies with 786,076 participants and found that compared to those who ate the least whole-grain foods, those who ate the most had a 16 percent decreased risk of all-cause mortality and an 18 percent decreased chance of dying from cardiovascular causes. The study also found that each 16-gram increase in whole grains people ate reduced mortality risk by 7 percent.[3]

That's all well and good in regard to whole-wheat grain foods, you might be thinking. *But what about the type of bread most of us often eat, white flour?*

White flour is not healthy, but having white flour on occasion is okay. Some foods like pizza are so great that having them from time to time arguably is good for our mental well-being. Also, when it comes to pizza, for instance, the tomato sauce is rich in powerful antioxidants such as lycopene. In addition, you're getting garlic, onion, basil, and other herbs and spices, all of which may help offset some of the negatives associated with white flour.

One of the tenets of this book is to enjoy life (we spend a whole chapter talking about the importance of being happy), so food with white flour, such as pizza or pasta or a great sandwich, is perfectly fine as a treat. Pasta, potatoes, and other good, complex carbs have actually been shown to help weight loss, because among other things, they fill people up and decrease cravings.[4]

That being said, many of the foods mentioned above often are better for us when made with high-quality whole-grain products. The problem is the quality of whole-grain products in the United States has been decimated by decades of industrial bread production that favored cheaper, easier-to-produce, and longer-lasting white flour.

—————

How can a nation be called great if its bread tastes like Kleenex?

—JULIA CHILD

—————

Though humans have been eating whole grains for longer than recorded history, white bread is an invention of the modern world.

Prehistoric humans chewed wheat berries and created some type of precursor to cereal with them. Ultimately, they learned that these berries could be pressed and pounded into a paste (flour), which when placed over a fire would harden into a flatbread. They later discovered (likely by accident) that when yeast was introduced to the crushed wheat berries, they could make leavened (raised) bread.

Because bread was such a reliable food source that could be stored for long periods, early civilizations, such as the ones in Mesopotamia and Egypt, were built on large-scale planting of wheat. Wheat also powered the most popular beverage of the day, beer.

Prior to the Industrial Revolution, early Americans enjoyed a rich variety of whole-grain bread types and flavors. That all changed in the 1800s when the steel roller mill was developed for flour production. This invention forever altered the way humans made and consumed wheat by enabling mass production of white flour.

Wheat grains have three primary parts: the bran, a nutrient-rich outer coating that has lots of fiber; the germ, which is the embryo of the wheat plant and provides flavor and aromatics to whole-wheat bread; and the endosperm, which provides nutrients to the germ and accounts for most of the grain's mass. For millennia, the various methods used to create flour still kept all three parts of the wheat grain together, but with roller mills used to produce flour, the endosperm is diminished and the germ and bran are discarded. This produces a less nutritious, less flavorful bread stripped of most of its healthy properties. It also produces a less oily bread that has a far longer shelf life than its whole-wheat counterparts.

Because of its uniformity and long shelf life, white bread became more popular and an unfortunate mainstay of Western diets. As the bread-producing process became even more industrialized in the 1900s and moved into factories, more gluten was added to the bread to improve its elasticity and uniformity.

Today's bread is generally whiter and less nutritious and has far more gluten in it than what our ancestors, and in many cases even our grandparents, ate. Only about 6 percent of the flour currently produced in the United States is whole wheat, and even some of that supposedly whole-wheat flour is suspect. Ferris Jabra noted in *The New York Times* that many so-called whole-wheat products are made from processed wheat that has had the oily germ and bran added back. The actual composition of the final product available to consumers is unclear, as is how the germ is added back without diminishing quality or shortening shelf life.

David Killilea, a nutrition scientist at the Children's Hospital Oakland Research Institute in California, says big mills might deactivate the living germ by steaming it or exposing it to gamma rays.[5]

Modern wheat is very different and likely less healthy than the ancient grains. Therefore it pays to seek out ancient varieties like einkorn, farro, and spelt.

Some theorize that the modified wheat and the change in bread production have created an uptick in gluten intolerance, though this notion is controversial. While there are people who do have gluten sensitivities, some adverse reactions may be incorrectly blamed on gluten. A 2011 study published in *The American Journal of Gastroenterology* looked at thirty-four people with irritable bowel syndrome. Some were given gluten-free pastries and others were given pastries with gluten. Because it was a double-blind study, neither the participants nor the researchers knew which pastries contained gluten. Most of those who ate the gluten pastries reported IBS symptoms, while most of those who ate the gluten-free muffins did not report pain.[6]

This study was widely hailed as proof of non-celiac gluten

intolerance, but as is true with many studies, you can't be too quick to take the results at face value. In a follow-up study, the same researchers found that gluten itself was probably not to blame. Instead, the problem arose from a group of foods known as FODMAPs, an acronym for what sounds like it might make a good song for Mary Poppins: fermentable oligosaccharides, disaccharides, monosaccharides, and polyols. FODMAPs include many, but not all, carbohydrates—they include high-fructose foods like apples, milk, ice cream, garlic, and onions. In the second study, researchers looked at thirty-seven volunteers who reported ill effects from gluten. When gluten and FODMAPs were removed from their diet, they didn't report any symptoms, and when gluten was reintroduced without FODMAPs, they still had no symptoms.[7]

We've found that some people just feel better when avoiding wheat, dairy, or sweets. Simply put, those people indeed should avoid those substances most of the time. People also should consider grinding their own wheat berries as needed, as this is by far the healthier route, and using different grains, not just modern wheat all the time, is a good idea. Durum wheat is great for pasta, and rye makes a dense and incredible bread. Also, ancient grains like einkorn may be enjoyed and well tolerated by people with some gluten sensitivities who have not been diagnosed with celiac disease.

On a summer's day in New York City, we're enjoying a slice of pizza at the original Patsy's Pizzeria in East Harlem. The quintessentially New York pie sold here is a thin-crust slice of paradise.

Although the pizza dough is made with white flour, it retains some of the dough-making artistry of old, with the right amount of crispness and chewiness, and of course, it has the delicious and nutritious lycopene-rich tomato sauce.

Farther downtown in New York City at Grand Central Terminal (a short walk from our Park Avenue office), there is Nordic-style rye bread offered for sale at the Great Northern Food Hall. The hall is owned by Claus Meyer, the founder of the legendary restaurant Noma in Copenhagen, whom *The New York Times* described as a "bread evangelist." He told the *Times* that "rugbrod [rye bread] is like wine in France or olive oil in Italy," and added, "It is more than food. It is history. It is culture, and agriculture."[8]

Biting into the rye bread he sells gives one a sense of bread's history and what it could be again in the future. Dark, dense, and wonderfully chewy, this rugbrod is rich with flavors most of us are not accustomed to in bread, but should become better acquainted with in our diets.

Thanks to the locavore movement, there are artisan bread makers across the country who are producing true whole-wheat bread that is not only more nutritious but more delicious than its white-flour counterparts. If you can't find a good bread maker near where you live, making your own is also a great option.

While Erik was growing up, our house was filled with the aroma of fresh-made whole-wheat bread, homemade whole-wheat pasta, and other whole-wheat products like cookies, waffles, and pancakes, all made from wheat berries just ground in a small grinder in the kitchen.

The bread was airy and rich with a crisp crust and soft interior, the pasta was as good as we've had anywhere, and the pancakes have yet to be equaled and have left us with a permanent dislike of white-flour pancakes.

If you're not accustomed to whole wheat and whole grains, you may need to retrain your taste buds. Think of it like craft beer versus light beer. Light beer is easier to drink, has less flavor overall and therefore less flavor to dislike, but once you develop a taste for IPAs, sours, stouts, and other craft beers, it's hard to go back to what then starts to feel like a watered-down beer.

Try to go to bakeries that either grind their own grains or get them freshly ground from local organic suppliers. Better yet, as suggested earlier, grind your own as needed and try baking some naturally fermented sourdough bread. If that's not possible, still go for 100 percent whole grain.

After visiting the Great Northern Food Hall, we gaze up at the clear, crisp fall sky above Grand Central and can't help but remember Ralph Waldo Emerson's words: "The sky is the daily bread of the eyes." We're thankful that we can break bread with good friends and family, and strive to be more tolerant of people and things, even the much-maligned gluten.

CHAPTER ELEVEN

BREAK-FAST, DIET LESS

■ ■ ■

Life, within doors, has few pleasanter prospects than
a neatly arranged and well-provisioned
breakfast table.

—NATHANIEL HAWTHORNE

IN BRIEF: Eating breakfast appears to be good for heart health and weight loss. So enjoy a natural, nutrient-rich breakfast instead of adopting fad diets, as they are mostly ineffective at keeping weight off. In addition, being ultra-skinny isn't necessarily healthier, and there are lots of fresh, natural, great-tasting foods that are also healthy.

We've got some good news and some bad news. The bad news is that most diets don't keep weight off in the long run. The good news is being slightly overweight may be healthier than being ultra-skinny, and eating big breakfasts might help us lose weight and be healthier. We're repeating that last part because it makes us happy: Eating breakfast is fun and can be good for us.

If you don't eat breakfast, that's okay too as long as you don't go loading up on high-calorie, low-nutrient foods later in the day. Researchers at Loma Linda University School of Public Health in California looked at the eating habits of 50,000 adults for a

2017 study. They found that those who ate their largest meals earlier in the day had a greater chance of having a lower body mass index (BMI), and breakfast eaters tended to weigh less than breakfast skippers. As the study concluded, "Our results suggest that in relatively healthy adults, eating less frequently, no snacking, consuming breakfast, and eating the largest meal in the morning may be effective methods for preventing long-term weight gain."[1]

This is only the latest research suggesting we should take the "fast" out of breakfast. Similar results were found in a small clinical trial at the Wolfson Medical Center in Tel Aviv. For the trial, dozens of obese women were put on 1,400-calorie-a-day diets that were identical, except the women were grouped by when they ate the majority of their calories. One group ate a 700-calorie meal for breakfast, 500 calories at lunch, and 200 calories for dinner; another group reversed this order. After twelve weeks, those who ate large breakfasts lost two and a half times as much as those who consumed large dinners (though both groups lost weight).[2]

The reasons behind this phenomenon are not fully understood, but our bodies seem to be better at producing insulin in the morning than in the evening, which means we might store more fat after an evening meal than after a morning meal.

As Dr. Satchidananda Panda, a professor at the Salk Institute for Biological Studies in San Diego, told *The New York Times*, "If you give a healthy individual a big bolus of glucose in the morning, the blood glucose might stay high one or two hours before coming back to normal. . . . You take that same normal healthy individual and give them the same bolus of glucose late at night, and now the pancreas is sleeping—literally—and cannot produce enough insulin, and blood glucose will stay high up to three hours." He added that this condition once was called "evening diabetes."[3]

The Loma Linda researchers also found an association between weight control and those who ate dinner earlier and therefore fasted longer during the evening. Those who had an eighteen- to nineteen-hour gap between their last meal of the day and breakfast the next morning had the lowest BMIs.

Eating more and earlier in the day (i.e., a big breakfast) might help extend this apparently helpful evening fast. A study conducted in mice found that those with unlimited access to a high-fat diet became obese and developed diabetes within nine to ten weeks, while another group of mice who ate high-fat foods for only eight hours a day did not become obese or diabetic even though they ate the same amount of calories as the all-day binge-ing mice.[4]

And the benefits of a hearty breakfast extend beyond weight loss.

A study published in the *Journal of the American College of Cardiology* in 2017 found middle-aged adults who regularly skip breakfast are more likely to have clogged arteries than those who regularly eat breakfast. For the study, researchers in Madrid examined a total of 4,052 volunteers, both male and female, who were free from cardiovascular or chronic kidney disease. Their results will make you want to dig out your grandmother's pancake recipe. Breakfast skippers (those who consumed only 5 percent of their daily energy intake in the morning) and low-energy breakfast eaters (who consumed between 5 to 20 percent of their energy intake in the morning) had greater frequencies of atherosclerosis—hardening and narrowing of the arteries—when compared to breakfast eaters (those who consumed 20 percent of their daily energy intake in the morning). In addition, cardiometabolic risk markers were more common among breakfast skippers and light morning eaters, as on average they had greater waist circumferences, higher BMIs, elevated blood pressures, elevated levels of blood lipids, and higher fasting glucose levels.

"People who regularly skip breakfast likely have an overall unhealthy lifestyle," said study author Valentin Fuster in a release, adding, "This study provides evidence that this is one bad habit people can proactively change to reduce their risk for heart disease."[5]

We assure you, the research cited thus far in this chapter has not been sponsored by a waffle company. That being said, there is some debate about the role of breakfast in the nutrition world, with some studies finding mixed weight loss results. But the evidence in favor of breakfast is significant enough that in 2017, the American Heart Association released a scientific statement encouraging the eating of a morning meal. In the statement, Marie-Pierre St-Onge, an associate professor of nutritional medicine at Columbia University in New York City, said, "Meal timing may affect health due to its impact on the body's internal clock. In animal studies, it appears that when animals receive food while in an inactive phase, such as when they are sleeping, their internal clocks are reset in a way that can alter nutrient metabolism, resulting in greater weight gain, insulin resistance and inflammation."

The statement also noted a connection "between eating breakfast and having lower heart disease risk factors. Studies have found people who eat breakfast daily are less likely to have high cholesterol and blood pressure, and people who skip breakfast—about 20 percent to 30 percent of U.S. adults—are more likely to be obese, have inadequate nutrition, show evidence of impaired glucose metabolism or be diagnosed with diabetes."[6]

Let food be thy medicine, and medicine be thy food.

—HIPPOCRATES

Now it's time to talk about those pesky diets. Diets often are a lot like cults. They're started by charismatic leaders, and successful ones attract fierce adherents who believe their way is the true path toward either divinity or weight loss.

The diet publishing and blogging industry seems to be ever expanding, with more books, websites, and weight loss columns published each year than anyone could possibly read—each claiming its method of reducing calories consumed is more effective than any other method for reducing calories. While reading has countless benefits, weight loss is not one of them.

In these books and articles we're encouraged to fast, detox, control our portions, and cleanse ourselves to health. But it doesn't take a statistician to tell you that despite our diet-obsessed culture, our collective waistline is expanding, and as a whole we're not ready for those wedding photographs.

So why aren't these diets working for most people?

It actually isn't so much that most diets don't work; it's that they don't work in the long run. If you follow most diets, you'll lose weight. However, we have an extra-large-sized caveat to that statement. Recent research shows that diets are essentially ineffective at keeping weight off.

One study of 278,982 people in the United Kingdom over a nine-year period found disturbingly few obese people could maintain weight loss over the course of the study: just 1 out of every 210 men studied and 1 out of every 124 women. "The probability of attaining normal weight or maintaining weight loss is low," the authors wrote. "Obesity treatment frameworks grounded in community-based weight management programs may be ineffective."[7]

This is a sobering study, but for those who have struggled to keep weight off, we've got something to cheer you up. Being a little overweight appears to be okay from a medical standpoint, and may even be beneficial. A recent study conducted at Copenhagen University Hospital in Denmark looked at more than 100,000 adults in that country and found those with an "overweight" BMI were more likely to live longer than those in the "obese," "healthy," or "underweight" categories.[8]

Another study coauthored by researchers at the University of California at Los Angeles and the University of California, Santa Barbara, discovered that the BMI index incorrectly labels more than 54 million Americans as "unhealthy," even though their blood pressure and blood work show they are healthy. The study found that close to half of Americans who are labeled "overweight" because of their BMI index are in fact healthy (47.4 percent, or 34.4 million people). An additional 19.8 million considered "obese" were healthy, while more than 30 percent of those with BMIs in the "normal" range, about 20.7 million people, were found to be unhealthy.[9]

While these studies go a long way toward discrediting the universal acceptance of BMI measurement, which is calculated by dividing a person's weight (in kilograms) by the square of their height (in meters), they don't actually prove that being overweight is healthier than being skinny. They just suggest it might not necessarily be less healthy. It is quite possible that as long as you exercise regularly, don't sit too long, and are a normal weight or even slightly overweight, you may even be a bit healthier than if you were emaciated or very skinny.

In one study of 4,900 adults, regular eating and having no history of dieting were associated with "successful weight maintenance in young women and men." As this study's coauthor, Ulla Kärkkäinen of the University of Helsinki, was quoted as saying in the *New York Post*: "In practice, people are encouraged to lose weight, whereas the results of our extensive population study indicate that losing weight is not an effective weight management method in the long run."[10]

A *New England Journal of Medicine* study found that "some foods—vegetables, nuts, fruits, and whole grains—were associated with less weight gain when consumption was actually increased . . . persons who eat more fruits, nuts, vegetables, and whole grains would gain less weight over time. Yogurt consumption was also associated with less weight gain in all three cohorts."[11] We heartily concur.

There's even better news coming out of the 90+ Study, a premier study of longevity examining the oldest of the old from the University of California, Irvine. Researchers from the 90+ Study have published many scientific papers in premier journals. Some of the major findings are that "people who drank moderate amounts of alcohol or coffee lived longer than those who abstained" and that "people who were overweight in their seventies lived longer than normal or underweight people did."[12]

There are hundreds upon hundreds of diet books; this is not one of them. So far no one we know has definitively shown how to effectively lose weight and also keep it off. So don't think you have to chase the latest diet craze, or be ultra-thin to be healthy. This doesn't mean you should try to become overweight. While being slightly overweight may not be as unhealthy as once thought, there is little question that being very overweight is decidedly unhealthy. There is also research suggesting systematic undereating is good for you and will help you live longer. However, current knowledge about weight and health trends should free you up to focus not on the temporary weight loss offered by fad diets, but rather on being healthier and happier in general.

We advocate living, working, and making a lifestyle out of being healthier. So stock up on primarily healthy foods, take a hike (literally), and enjoy life more. In addition to enjoying the good vices we've talked about in this book, make sure to eat lots of fruits and vegetables, including garlic and onions and fermented foods. If you eat foods that look like they grew up from, walked on, swam across, or flew above the earth, that food is probably pretty good for you. If you look at the food and have no idea whether it came from a 3-D printer or the moon, we advise more caution.

Speaking of diet fads, as we discuss at length in the chapter on fat-free products, these foods are not really effective at facilitating either weight loss or better health. As mentioned in the sugar chapter, diet soda is bad for your health and weight maintenance. So avoid those supposed "diet" products and remember that healthy eating often is wonderfully delicious eating. To remind our readers of this, we've developed a simple meal plan we call the VIP Non-Diet Diet that combines three different effective nutritional lifestyles. In this loose plan, the vegetarian plant- and grain-based diet is combined with the primal ancient and unprocessed food diet (a diet that can include grass-fed and -finished meat and raw and fermented dairy), and the rich flavors and varied cuisine of the international/Mediterranean diet.

To better understand how to implement this, picture three overlapping circles with the foods allowed in each diet/meal plan in each circle.

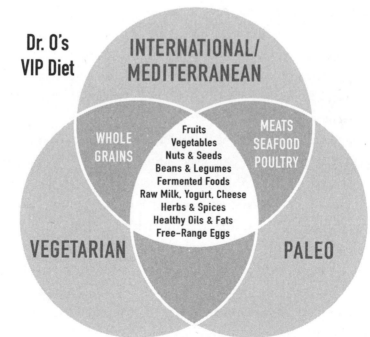

Dr. O's VIP Diet

INTERNATIONAL/ MEDITERRANEAN

WHOLE GRAINS

Fruits
Vegetables
Nuts & Seeds
Beans & Legumes
Fermented Foods
Raw Milk, Yogurt, Cheese
Herbs & Spices
Healthy Oils & Fats
Free-Range Eggs

MEATS SEAFOOD POULTRY

VEGETARIAN

PALEO

The places where all three diets intersect are often the healthiest. For example, fruits and vegetables (fermented and otherwise) are permitted in each diet, as are beans and legumes, nuts and seeds, healthy oils and fats, free-range eggs (they are vegetarian, though not vegan), dairy yogurt and cheese. These foods are excellent for you and should be consumed in greater abundance, barring any specific allergies. Each person is an individual with individual health and nutritional needs. As such, foods found in only one or two of the three circles still can be a healthy part of an individual nutrition plan.

It's hard to overstate how healthy some of the foods available on this plan are, especially the ones that appear in all three spheres. Garlic, for instance, has a laundry list of health benefits, like vitamin C, vitamin B_6, and manganese, to mention only a few. In addition, garlic can decrease the length of the common cold, lower blood pressure, improve cholesterol levels, and fight infection. We've noticed that many long-lived individuals consume large quantities of garlic and other similarly spicy vegetables like onions and peppers.

In general, do not doubt that what you eat can have as great an effect as medication. One major clinical trial of 7,447 people found switching to a Mediterranean diet could reduce about 30 percent of heart attacks, strokes, and all deaths from heart disease for people at high risk. This is comparable to the results when using prescribed statins. The study characterized the Mediterranean diet as one with "a high intake of olive oil, fruits, nuts, vegetables, and cereals; a moderate intake of fish and poultry; a low intake of dairy products, red meat, processed meats, and sweets; and wine in moderation, consumed with meals."[13]

When combining the elements of an international/Mediterranean diet with primal and vegetarian diets, we don't recommend specific amounts because our VIP nutritional plan isn't really a diet. Most diet rules are arbitrary and too hard for most of us to follow for significant lengths of time. The trick here is enjoying what you eat, not overeating, and making sure it makes you feel great, not guilty or bad. As for all those diet books gathering dust on your shelf, they probably aren't doing you any good healthwise, but hey, maybe you can strap them together and use them in place of weights. Though, as we discuss in the next chapter, extreme exercise can sometimes be as overrated as extreme dieting.

CHAPTER TWELVE

SKIP TO THE GYM

■ ■ ■

An early-morning walk is a blessing for the whole day.
—HENRY DAVID THOREAU

Eating alone will not keep a man well;
he must also take exercise.
—HIPPOCRATES

IN BRIEF: While exercise is very important, extreme exercise might be overrated. Research suggests moderate exercisers can be at least as healthy, and sometimes even healthier, as those who exercise excessively, and the link between weight loss and intense workouts may be overestimated. Little things, like a brisk short walk or a standing desk, can make a big difference. Exercise is extremely healthy, and not exercising is not a good idea, so just do it, but don't feel compelled to overdo it. Get off your duff throughout the day. Find physical activities you enjoy, like walking, jogging, running, or bicycling; then do one several times a week for fun.

It's time for the lazy to proudly stand . . . er . . . raise their fists in the air in a slow, not overly strenuous show of solidarity. A growing—but not overly ripped—body of research has found that although exercise has health benefits, certain levels of extreme exercise do not add to your overall well-being and may even hinder it.

So skip your predawn decathlon, and sit back and enjoy some guilt-free relaxation as we make a high-energy case for the benefits of moderate-energy workouts. In 2015, *Circulation*, a journal of the American Heart Association, published one of the biggest studies to look at the effects of too much exercise, which they defined as any type of exercise that causes sweating or a fast heartbeat engaged in more than two to three times a week. The results were heart-stopping—sometimes literally. Researchers looked at 1.1 million women age fifty to sixty-four and tracked their cardiovascular health for nine years.

To nobody's surprise, the study showed that exercise was indeed good for you, *but only to a point.* Moderate exercisers experienced dramatically fewer adverse vascular events (any health complications affecting the circulatory system) compared to nonexercisers. At four to seven strenuous sessions a week, exercisers experienced *increased* adverse vascular effects. Even when it came to nonstrenuous exercise, including gardening and housework, four to six days a week was best, and seven days a week was associated with a rise in vascular troubles.[1]

Counterintuitive as it may sound, this study is in keeping with other research indicating diminishing returns on extreme exercise for men and women. A 2018 study in the *American Journal of Preventive Medicine* found that on exercise days, people "had more physical activity energy expenditure, but because of reductions in other activities, only about half of the energy expended during exercise was added to total daily physical activity energy expenditure."[2]

An earlier report in the *Journal of the American College of Cardiology* found that runners who pounded the pavement too often and too strenuously saw rapid declines in benefits and even adverse effects from the extreme exercise. The study of 1,098 healthy joggers and 3,950 healthy non-joggers in Denmark over a twelve-year period concluded that too little running or too much running was linked to higher rates of death.[3]

In an article about the study, *Time* magazine declared the proper level of exercise was a Goldilocks amount, one just right to maintain heart health, burn calories, and keep blood sugar levels under control, but according to the researchers behind this study, "that sweet spot is closer to the 'less' side of the curve than the 'more' side."[4]

The scientists concluded that the ideal pace to jog was about five miles per hour and that it was best to jog about three times per week. That's a decent amount of movement, but it's certainly not the regimen marathon victories are made of. In general, runners, including long-distance runners, are often much healthier than those who are sedentary. So don't hesitate to not only skip but bike or run to the gym as well.

We want to make something crystal clear before we go forward: For every study showing a possible risk from strenuous exercise, there are dozens showing the importance of exercise overall. The takeaway from this chapter is that people need not engage in extreme exercise for health. Moderate, more doable exercise for many is full of health benefits. Sitting for long periods of time is unhealthy, but when it comes to exercise, a little bit can go a long way.

Researchers have begun looking at micro-workouts—short, intense exercises with positive results. A group of fourteen sedentary men and women were studied while engaging in what's been called the one-minute workout. Participants spent ten minutes three times a week on stationary bikes. They would warm up by cycling slowly for two minutes, bike as hard they could for twenty-second intervals, followed by two minutes of slower cycling, until they had biked fast for a total of a minute. Then they'd cool down for three minutes. After six weeks, participants had improved their endurance by about 12 percent and had better blood work.[5]

Beyond short bursts of intense activity, not being sedentary is just as important. Many recent studies have sung the praises of standing desks. Spending some of the workday pacing or walking in place or on a treadmill at your desk, rather than sitting at it, promotes movement and limits our time sitting. This is all good, since long durations of uninterrupted sitting have been linked to an increased chance of death.[6]

When it comes to exercise, walking is often wrongly overlooked as not intense enough. Walking is one of our favorite forms of exercise and offers a plethora of health benefits. The effect of regular short walks adds up, helping us burn calories and improve overall health. Try to take walks during your lunch break or suggest a "walking meeting" instead of the standard conference room meeting. Look for the parking space farthest from your destination and take the stairs instead of the elevator when you can. Little things add up. Hiking in the woods offers even more benefits.

Walking also can improve our mental health and help us relax. The Japanese practice of "forest bathing" is increasingly popular in the United States. The idea behind the practice is that instead of just hiking, people go outside and enjoy nature in a mindful, relaxed manner. Spending time in the forest this way may have a profound effect. As the Association of Nature and Forest Therapy points out, "Physical activity in the form of a 40-minute walk in the forest" has been "associated with improved mood and feelings of health and robustness." In "a 2007 study, men taking two-hour walks in the woods over a two-day period exhibited a 50 percent increase in levels of natural killer cells—the body's disease fighting agents." One 2008 study of thirteen female nurses on a three-day forest-bathing trip found "the trip produced anti-cancer proteins and benefits lasting more than 7 days after the trip."[7]

More research is needed, since the extent of the benefits is unclear, as is the role of the forest itself. Some believe, for example, that the natural chemicals secreted by evergreen trees, collectively called phytoncides, are specifically helping the immune system. In that case, how much nature would be needed to enjoy the benefits of forest bathing? Would a park work? At this time we don't know. But it seems a safe bet to us that spending time outside in nature, or as close to nature as we can get if we live in a city, is a good idea. Whenever you can, walk barefoot on the beach, grass, or forest paths. Look, smell, and feel the natural world around you.

Now it's time to address the 800-pound-but-on-a-wheat-free-diet gorilla in the room—weight loss. Let's be honest, when it comes to exercise, especially excessive exercise, most of us are more concerned with appearance than health. But despite what the people touting the latest over-the-top intense exercise regime would lead you to believe, exercise and weight loss appear only casually linked—if they were people, they would be Facebook friends but wouldn't really know why.

In a study published in *Population Health Metrics* in 2013, researchers found that physical activity increased between 2001 and 2009, particularly in Kentucky, Georgia, and Florida, but the rise in exercise was matched by an increase in obesity in nearly every county the researchers studied, even with controls for changing rates in poverty, unemployment, and other metrics.[8]

A possible reason exercise doesn't have as big an effect on weight loss as we believe it should is that as exercise burns calories, it can increase our appetites, causing us to eat more. We also might rationalize eating more after we exercise—you know, the whole "I went to the gym and exercised for eight minutes, so now I'm going to enjoy that bacon burger with eighteen pounds of fries on the side."

When we engage in this type of thinking, we often tip the caloric scale in the wrong direction. As Aseem Malhotra, a cardiologist, wrote in *The Washington Post*, "If you exercise for the purpose of burning calories, you get a very low return on investment: You would have to walk for more than 45 minutes to burn off the 300 calories from eating just three cookies."

On top of that, Malhotra argues that the notion that physical activity increases our metabolism, so our bodies consume calories at a quicker rate, is exaggerated. He points to a 2012 study where anthropologists measured the daily physical activity, metabolic rates, and energy expenditure of people in a hunter-gatherer tribe in Tanzania, and compared the results to the average Westerner.

The Tanzanians were, as expected, much more physically active, but their metabolic rates were similar to their more sedentary counterparts in the West. The other problem with extreme exercise regimes is that even if they're working to keep weight down, they often come to abrupt ends and are followed by rapid and unhealthy weight gain.[9]

Though couch potatoes may be jumping for joy—except of course that would involve, you know, getting off the couch and exerting themselves—this doesn't mean you should trade the treadmill for the sofa. Exercise overwhelmingly has been shown to be very healthy for most people, whereas prolonged sitting is decidedly very, very unhealthy. Interestingly, this even seems to be true for newborn infants, who often spend way too much time sitting on their back in car seats or strollers.[10]

Like so much else in this book, the secret when it comes to exercise is, well, common sense. It might not always lead to significant weight loss by itself, but paired with a nonextreme diet, it will make you a lot healthier. Don't feel guilty because you're not jumping on an exercise bike seven days a week and have yet to set any land speed records. Instead of driving to the gym, take a long walk to the neighborhood coffeehouse. When it comes to health, it appears slow and steady (or intervals of slow and steady alternating with short fast bursts) may actually win the race.

CHAPTER THIRTEEN

LET THE SUNSHINE IN

■ ■ ■

"My son, I caution you to keep the middle way,
for if your pinions dip too low the waters
may impede your flight; and if they soar
too high the sun may scorch them. Fly midway.
Gaze not at the boundless sky."
—DAEDALUS TO HIS SON, ICARUS,
OVID'S *METAMORPHOSES*

IN BRIEF: Soak up the sun in moderation. The sun's rays are a natural source of vitamin D and can boost the immune system and provide a host of health benefits. Too little sunlight puts us at risk for a variety of diseases, including cancer, and can decrease life expectancy. While it is certainly true that overexposure to the sun can cause skin cancer, too little sunlight can be unhealthy as well.

Don't fly too close to the sun. That's what the mythical Greek inventor Daedalus warned his son, Icarus. Daedalus had fashioned two sets of wings for himself and Icarus out of feathers and wax in order for the pair to escape the island of Crete, where they were held captive. Icarus was told that if he got too near the sun, the wax holding the feathers together would melt.

Despite this warning, mesmerized by the joy of flight, Icarus flew too close to the sun. As predicted, the wax holding his wings together melted and he fell to his death. For centuries, the story has served as cautionary tale, a warning against the dangers of arrogance. But there's a part of the myth we tend to forget: Icarus also was warned against timidity and too much caution, and told if he played it too safe and flew too close to the ocean, the sea's dampness would cause the wings' feathers to sag. To survive, Icarus needed to find the happy medium between the sun and the water.

This is a great metaphor for moderation in general, and when it comes to exposing our skin to the sun, it can be taken almost literally. We need sunlight physically and emotionally. When our skin is hit by direct sunlight, it forms vitamin D, thanks to the photosynthetic-like reaction caused by ultraviolet (UV) radiation. If we are too timid and avoid or block all sun, we greatly increase our chances of a vitamin D deficiency, which can increase our risk for a host of life-threatening ailments. On the other hand, if we're overconfident and get too much sun, we increase our chances of skin cancer.

Most medical advice has been focused on artificially blocking the sun, treating it exclusively as a dangerous and sometimes deadly side effect of the joys of summer. Recent evidence, however, suggests that hiding completely from the sun may be potentially even more injurious to our health.

According to one 2008 study based on World Health Organization data, harmful ultraviolet radiation (UVR) exposure from the sun is only "a minor contributor to the world's disease burden." Researchers assess the risk of UVR exposure by measuring disability-adjusted life years (DALYs), which tracks the number of years that people lose because of ill health, disability, or premature death from disease. UVR exposure accounts for only an "annual loss of 1.6 million DALYs; i.e., 0.1% of the total global disease burden." This pales (pun very much intended) in comparison to the "markedly larger annual disease burden, [of] 3.3 billion DALYs, [that] might result from reduction in global UVR exposure to very low levels."[1]

A study published in 2016 in the *Journal of Internal Medicine* proclaimed "avoidance of sun exposure is a risk factor for death of a similar magnitude as smoking." For the study, researchers looked at 29,518 Swedish women. They found that although those who got sunlight had an increased risk of skin cancer, they had a decreased risk of death overall.[2]

According to the most recent sun-protection recommendations of the Centers for Disease Control and Prevention, "The sun's ultraviolet (UV) rays can damage your skin in as little as 15 minutes." People are encouraged, when possible, to stay in the shade, and even when in the shade to cover up with "long-sleeved shirts" and "long pants and skirts." It's also recommended they wear "a hat with a brim all the way around" to shade their "face, ears and the back of [their] neck."

On the off chance that a ray of sunlight, despite all these precautions, might slip through and hit uncovered skin, the CDC also advises people to "put on broad spectrum sunscreen with at least SPF 15 before you go outside, even on slightly cloudy or cool days."[3]

This advice will indeed prevent some skin cancers and might work well for vampires, but is somewhat impractical for most warm-blooded, non-undead human beings. Those who follow the advice thoroughly will be largely free of the dangers posed by the sun, which is thought to be the cause of more than 90 percent of skin cancer cases, but also will have missed out on the benefits of sunlight.

In the past, sunscreen has sometimes done more harm than good, as many sunscreens did not (and many still don't) block all types of potentially cancer-causing UV rays. You are better off using naturally light, breathable, sun-protective clothing, hats, and umbrellas, but if you do wear sunscreen, bear in mind that those that have the most broad spectrum and have more zinc oxide may be more effective. People who use ineffective sunscreen may think they are protected and stay in the sun longer, possibly burning and not knowing it while increasing their risk of cancer. At the same time, ineffective sunscreen often blocks rays that would help the skin produce vitamin D, therefore possibly eliminating much of the benefit of being in the sun. In addition, chemicals contained in many sunscreens can be harmful to the environment. Hawaii banned certain sunscreens because chemicals within them were harming ocean ecosystems.

As noted earlier, sunlight is an important source of vitamin D. When it comes to our collective vitamin D levels, the news is as sobering as a rain forecast on a holiday weekend. By some estimates, about 50 percent of people don't have sufficient levels of vitamin D, and as many as 1 billion people suffer from a vitamin D deficiency worldwide.

Writing for the *Journal of Pharmacology & Pharmacotherapeutics* in 2012, Rathish Nair and Arun Maseeh call this vitamin D deficiency a "pandemic" (a global disease) and said "reduced outdoor activities" were among the lifestyle changes to blame.[4]

Researchers in Norway studied 115,096 cases of breast, colon, and prostate cancer diagnosed between 1964 and 1992 and found that those who received a cancer diagnosis in the summer and fall, the seasons when people have the highest levels of vitamin D, had a lower risk of cancer death—suggesting that a high level of vitamin D_3 at the time of diagnosis, and thus during cancer treatment, may improve a person's prognosis.[5]

It's not just vitamin D production that the sun is facilitating. Scientists at Georgetown University recently found that sunlight activates immune system cells, called T cells, causing them to move faster and be more effective, thus boosting the immune system's strength. Sunlight seems to be to T cells what steroids are to professional athletes, minus the negative side effects and 500-foot monster home runs, of course.[6]

As we mentioned in the sleep chapter, adequate sunlight can be vital when it comes to getting enough shut-eye. According to a study published in the *Journal of Clinical Sleep Medicine* in 2014, office workers in workspaces with more windows and natural sunlight enjoyed longer, better-quality sleep than those who worked in windowless offices. The study was small—only forty-nine people—but it had powerful results.

Not only did the workers with access to windows and sun enjoy an average of forty-six more minutes of sleep per night, they also reported a better quality of life and more physical activity. In other words, the stuffy, windowless offices too many of us toil away in today might be viewed by future generations with the same disapproval we now view the deplorable treatment of mine workers in the past.[7]

Speaking of the relationship between sleeping and sunlight,

exposure to early morning sunlight can help reset our circadian rhythms and seems to increase overall sleep by keeping us more in tune with natural day-and-night cycles. And watching the sunrise and/or sunset regularly can be a fun and beneficial way to improve health and well-being.[8]

So don't hide completely from the light. Get outside, take a walk, and smell the roses.

Just ten minutes of sunlight a few times a week will provide more than just physical benefits. Sunlight can decrease symptoms of depression, help improve bone density, and even help treat conditions such as arthritis and irritable bowel syndrome (IBS).

Those who live in colder climates with less direct overhead sunlight in the winter tend to suffer more from seasonal depression or seasonal affective disorder (SAD).

Henry Lindlahr, known as the father of modern naturopathic medicine, would recommend that patients air-bathe in natural daylight even in winter by walking completely naked in the garden in front of their rooms. Advice that might indeed be good for your health, but that will almost certainly lower your standing with your neighbors.

In northern regions above the 37th parallel, even when you do everything right, you often can't get enough vitamin D in the winter because the angle at which the sun is shining on the earth doesn't allow for enough sunlight exposure. When the sun's angle is so low that your shadow is taller than you, it's especially important to try to supplement your vitamin D with vitamin-rich foods such as salmon, mackerel, sardines, and natural vitamin D_3 supplements.

Unfortunately, due in part to our propensity to pollute the earth, sea, and air, and damage the ozone layer (the area within the stratosphere that helps shield the earth and us from potentially harmful UV radiation), too much sun too quickly can lead to an increase in our chances of skin cancer. To avoid this type of potentially dangerous overexposure, cover up with loose clothing, hats, umbrellas, and natural shade to shield yourself from the sun when necessary, starting with just a few minutes of exposure a day at first, so you gradually build up exposure and tan, rather than burn. Don't fear the sun, but don't get burned either.

Remember the tale of Icarus and his father's unheeded advice. Don't be arrogant and "fly" too close to the sun, but don't be so timid you hide from it entirely. That, too, can be dangerous and a whole lot less fun. As Oscar Wilde wrote:

Never regret thy fall
O Icarus of the fearless flight
For the greatest tragedy of them all
Is never to feel the burning light.

CHAPTER FOURTEEN

EAT OLD (FERMENTED) FOOD

■ ■ ■

It takes a sour woman to make a good pickle.
—MICHAEL CHABON,
THE YIDDISH POLICEMEN'S UNION

It is not sufficient, he emphasized,
to colour (colorare) the mind with wisdom;
it must be pickled (macerare) in it, as it were, soaked
in it (inficere), and entirely transformed by it.
—PETER SLOTERDIJK, *YOU MUST CHANGE YOUR LIFE*

IN BRIEF: Fermented foods such as pickles, sauerkraut, and other fermented vegetables and homemade yogurts are rich in nutrients and help power our microbiome with a variety of good bacteria, helping to reduce digestive issues and ward off a host of other health conditions.

Growing up in Brooklyn, Harry would run around the corner to the local appetizing store. These legendary delis and bagel shops, which are part of New York City lore, featured giant wooden barrels filled with pickled cucumbers, the quintessential companion to any deli sandwich. You could just reach into the barrels, grabbing incredibly delicious, naturally fermented pickles.

The pickling process not only preserved the cucumber and

gave it that delightful tartness but also helped turn it into a "superfood" that should be a large part of most people's diets. That's because when it comes to our health, being in a pickle is a good thing.

Humans have been fermenting food and drink for thousands of years, but it is only recently that we've begun to understand the process, at least a little bit. Broadly speaking, fermentation is the chemical breakdown of molecules such as glucose by bacteria, yeasts, or other microorganisms. It has been happening naturally for untold millennia and under the direction of humans for culinary purposes for at least ten thousand years, when the first alcoholic beverages we have evidence of were produced. It wasn't until the mid-1800s that we began to understand the invisible forces—the yeast and other microorganisms—that power the process of fermentation. Much of this new understanding came thanks to Louis Pasteur, the famed French chemist and biologist.

These tiny organisms, invisible to the naked eye, also play an active role in our health. Billions of bacteria are present within our bodies at all times and make up what is called the microbiome. This complex ecosystem plays a key role in our digestion and overall health in ways that we are only just beginning to understand. An unhealthy microbiome might be linked to autism, various emotional disorders, and a wide range of other conditions and illnesses. Consuming fermented food may help keep our microbiome in good working order.

We've already talked about the joys and potential health benefits of various fermented beverages (alcohols) in previous chapters; here we'll look at the fermentation process when applied to fruits and vegetables and explain why eating real pickles is good for your health.

In wine, spirits, and beer, fermentation occurs when yeast breaks down sugars (found in grapes and other fruits and grains) into alcohol. When it comes to fermented foods, the most common type of fermentation is lacto-fermentation, which does not, as the name might imply, have anything to do with either milk or lactation.

Lacto refers to lactobacillus, a species of bacteria found on the surface of many plants and in the gastrointestinal and genitourinary tracts of humans and other animals. During the process of fermentation, lactobacillus converts sugars into lactic acid, giving fermented foods their signature sour flavors. Lactobacillus also is used as a souring agent in many sour beers and is one of the bacteria used to sour yogurt. In addition to creating this delicious tartness, lactic acid is a natural preservative that prevents the growth of harmful bacteria, which extends the life of various foods. At the same time, the process preserves vitamin and enzyme levels and can provide our bodies with healthy bacteria.

In fact, fermented vegetables are one of nature's incredible health secrets. As mentioned earlier, the process takes normally incredibly healthy foods like vegetables and supercharges them. Fermented vegetables are more easily digested and can replenish and nourish the good bacteria in your gut.

Unsweetened natural whole-milk yogurt also is a superfood nutriment that is easily digested and loaded with probiotic live cultures and important vitamins and minerals like calcium, potassium, B_5, B_{12}, riboflavin, and of course, protein.

We have seen so many patients improve by simply eating

naturally fermented homemade yogurt and various fermented vegetables. In particular, many patients with gastrointestinal disorders, including irritable bowel syndrome and inflammatory bowel disease, have seen dramatic improvements after adding lots of fermented foods to their diet.

In 2016, a paper in *Current Opinion in Biotechnology* noted that "although only a limited number of clinical studies on fermented foods have been performed, there is evidence that these foods provide health benefits well beyond the starting food materials."[1]

In 2014, researchers argued in the *Journal of Physiological Anthropology* that "fermented foods may be particularly relevant to the emerging research linking traditional dietary practices and positive mental health." They added, "The extent to which traditional dietary items may mitigate inflammation and oxidative stress may be controlled, at least to some degree, by microbiota. It is our contention that properly controlled fermentation may often amplify the specific nutrient and phytochemical content of foods, the ultimate value of which may be associated with mental health; furthermore, we also argue that the microbes (for example, Lactobacillus and Bifidobacteria species) associated with fermented foods may also influence brain health via direct and indirect pathways."[2]

Some of this research yields evidence that those who consumed more traditional diets had better mental health and a decreased chance of suffering from depression. One study looked at 1,046 women age twenty to ninety-three, randomly selected from the population, and found that after adjustments for age, social and economic status, education, and health behaviors, "a 'traditional' dietary pattern characterized by vegetables, fruit, meat, fish and whole grains was associated with lower odds for major depression or dysthymia and for anxiety disorders."[3]

A separate study conducted in Spain looked at more than ten thousand adults and found that those who followed a Mediterranean diet were less likely to develop depressive disorders. This makes sense, as the diet is thought to reduce adverse inflammatory and vascular processes, which are considered risk factors in clinical depression.[4]

Though the last two studies mentioned above did not look at fermented foods in particular, traditional cultures historically consume large amounts of fermented foods, a practice that began as a necessity, since refrigeration is a relatively recent invention.

Unfortunately, not all fermented foods are created equal. Modern mass-produced sauerkraut and pickles offered at supermarkets are too often pickled or preserved in vinegar with added sugar and preservatives, or they might not be fermented at all. As a result, they may not contain all the good bacteria or be as healthy as the traditional pickles, sauerkraut, and other fermented foods mentioned above.

Thanks to the renewed interest in more natural diets, there has been a resurgence in traditionally fermented foods. Therefore delicious pickles and sauerkraut, as well as many other naturally fermented vegetables, are available at many farmers' markets and grocery stores. Ask for natural lactic-acid-fermented vegetables.

If you can't find high-quality fermented vegetables or just want to experiment with the world of fermentation, the process is easy to do in your own kitchen. You can pickle almost any vegetable; it doesn't have to be cucumbers. You can ferment beans, string beans, broccoli, cauliflower, and many other vegetables in hardly any time at all.

If possible, it's best to make your own yogurt from raw unhomogenized milk. When purchasing yogurt, look for whole-milk yogurt from pasture-raised cows.

Once you've found a good source of regular fermented foods, enjoy them with a fermented beverage. Kombucha is a popular fermented tea that traditionally is nonalcoholic. Beer and hard apple cider are great fermented beverages, and sour beers, as mentioned earlier, are often made with wild yeasts and lactobacillus bacteria the same way yogurt is, and like yogurt, they potentially can improve gut health.

Modern-day people would do well to follow in the footsteps of their ancestors and consume more fermented foods. Try to add that pickle, fermented vegetable, or yogurt to almost any meal, and you might just be healthier. And if it's as good as the pickles we used to enjoy in Brooklyn, you'll be a whole lot happier. Trust your gut and help it at the same time by eating and drinking delicious fermented foods.

CHAPTER FIFTEEN

BREASTFEEDING IS BEST FEEDING

. . .

I lost most of my weight from breastfeeding
and I encourage women to do it;
it's just so good for the baby and good for yourself.
—BEYONCÉ

IN BRIEF: Breastfeeding is healthy for babies, decreasing their illnesses and strengthening their immune systems. It also is good for mothers.

Why do we include breastfeeding as a good vice? As we discuss in greater detail later, the majority of women do not follow the UN World Health Organization's basic recommendation to breastfeed exclusively for at least six months. We think they should.

For grown-ups, breastfeeding might sound like the opposite of a vice, but for babies, it's the quintessential good vice—something they naturally love that also is good for them.

For decades, however, mother's milk was denied far too many infants. Breastfeeding started to fall out of favor at the beginning of the twentieth century, especially in North America. Many both in and outside the medical community viewed it as a hindrance, an unseemly and unnecessary practice. Members of the baby boomer generation often were raised on formula, which, despite advertisements to the contrary, is not as healthy as breast milk.

The use of formula spread in part because formula companies aggressively marketed their products to mothers and medical professionals across the globe. "In exchange for handing out 'discharge packs' of formula, hospitals received freebies like formula and baby bottles," according to a *Business Insider* article.[1] A 1982 report in *New Internationalist* recounted these marketing tactics, noting "the most insidious of these is a free architectural service to hospitals which are building or renovating facilities for newborn care. . . . Baby milk companies spend untold millions of dollars subsidizing office furnishings, research projects, gifts, conferences, publications and travel junkets of the medical profession."[2]

Today the medical community is unequivocal in its stance that for healthy mothers, breastfeeding is indeed the best feeding. The American Academy of Pediatrics recommends that breastfeeding continue for at least twelve months after birth, and for as long as mother and baby desire thereafter. The World Health Organization (WHO) recommends continued breastfeeding up to two years of age and beyond.[3]

Sadly, as we will see, the majority of mothers do not follow this good advice.

As *Time* magazine reported in 2015, "Breast milk is a live substance full of immune-promoting and anti-inflammatory compounds, helping develop the immune system and a healthy microbiome." The article added, "Baby formula, on the other hand, also seems to change gut microbes, but not for the better: research shows that breast-fed babies have more natural-killer cells—a type of immune cell that targets and destroys cancer cells—than children fed with formula," and that there "are animal studies finding that breast milk contains stem cells that may be similar to embryonic stem cells, meaning they can change inside an infant's body and perform where they're needed."[4,5]

As microbiome researchers Jack Gilbert and Rob Knight note in their book *Dirt Is Good*, "Many studies show that breast-fed infants have better health outcomes than non-breast-fed infants—fewer ear infections, colds and bouts of diarrhea. They also have stronger immune systems, score higher in IQ tests, and may be less prone to obesity than other babies."

Breast milk is so healthy in large part because it provides needed nutrients to the microbes in the developing gut of infants. "A key ingredient is a menu of complex sugars (called oligosaccharides), and this is where humans stand out," Gilbert and Knight write. "The milk of cows, goats, sheep, and pigs contains oligosaccharide concentrations that are a hundred to a thousand times lower than human milk."

There also are benefits for mothers who breastfeed, ranging "from slimming down more rapidly to release of oxytocin that assists in bonding with your baby, to reduced risks of some kinds of cancers."[6]

Studies have shown that breastfeeding, especially for longer periods, helps reduce the risk of breast cancer and cancer in general in mothers. One of the latest studies supporting this reduction in risk was released in May 2017 by the World Cancer Research Fund International, and was based on a mammoth analysis of 119 global studies examining a total of 12 million women and more than 260,000 cases of breast cancer.[7] The study confirmed that breastfeeding significantly reduced the risk of breast cancer. Susannah Brown, senior science program manager at the World Cancer Research Fund International, wrote: "We recommend that mothers breast-feed infants exclusively (no other food or drink) for the first six months. . . . This recommendation is in line with the WHO recommendations on breastfeeding and U.N. Global Strategy on Infant and Young Child Feeding."[8]

Breastfeeding can help prevent cancer in children as well. One meta-analysis of eighteen studies found that breastfeeding was associated with as much as a 19 percent lower risk for childhood leukemia when compared to children who had never been breast-fed or were breastfed for shorter periods.[9]

Brown and the World Cancer Research Fund International found that "breast-fed children are less likely to be overweight or obese in adult life." This in turn diminished the risk of several types of cancer.[10]

In short, breast milk is nature's perfect food. All the benefits of and advice for facilitating breastfeeding are too numerous for us to go into in this chapter. There is, however, an abundance of information available from many reliable organizations. One of the oldest and most respected of these is La Leche League, an international organization devoted to helping mothers breastfeed.

Despite being almost universally recognized as something that is good for babies, breastfeeding is still difficult for many mothers because of societal taboos against it. It is frowned upon, if not outright forbidden, in most public places. These policies, regardless of their intentions, effectively stigmatize motherhood and make it difficult, and in some cases impossible, for mothers to give their babies the best possible source of sustenance.

At one university where we taught, the employee handbook included policies that said breastfeeding must be performed within designated "breastfeeding rooms." While these rooms were framed as an amenity, the message was clear: They were not merely spots for mothers looking for privacy, they were the *only* places breastfeeding was permitted on campus.

This policy didn't present any problems for most students or teachers, but a mother bringing a child to work or school, or pumping for a baby at home, should not have to be segregated in order to provide the healthiest food for her child. Imagine if we handled feeding children fruits or vegetables the same way!

These attitudes, plus other misinformed notions, have led to our current situation where a majority of babies are not breastfed as long as is recommended by the American Academy of Pediatrics or the World Health Organization. According to the most recent reports, while 81 percent of mothers start out breastfeeding, only 51 percent were still breastfeeding at six months and less than a third (30.7 percent) were still breastfeeding at 12 months.[11]

In addition, 70 percent of women do not follow the WHO recommendation to breastfeed exclusively (meaning no other food or drink) for at least six months. According to WHO, "Breastfeeding is an unequalled way of providing ideal food for the healthy growth and development of infants; it is also an integral part of the reproductive process with important implications for the health of mothers. Review of evidence has shown that, on a population basis, exclusive breast-feeding for six months is the optimal way of feeding infants."

To sustain this six-month period of exclusive breastfeeding, the WHO recommends:

- Initiation of breastfeeding within the first hour of life

- Exclusive breastfeeding—that means the infant receives only breast milk without any additional food or drink, not even water

- Breastfeeding on demand—that is as often as the child wants, day and night

- No use of bottles, teats, or pacifiers[12]

Breastfeeding, carrying, and not letting babies cry themselves to sleep are activities we are passionate about. We suggest all expectant mothers read Jean Liedloff's book *The Continuum Concept* and visit the Liedloff Continuum Network website, at www .continuum-concept.org.

Right about now some readers might be asking: What about mothers who are physically unable to breastfeed? In those rare cases, we advise women to not worry and instead consult with a naturopathic physician or other health-care provider. However, if it's a matter of scheduling and time, we suggest doing what you can to prioritize this healthy practice for you and your baby.

Some mothers work in environments that don't provide adequate resources for breastfeeding. If that's you, once again, we advise giving your boss a copy of this book with this chapter bookmarked. People, male and female, are afraid of angry moms, and when it comes to breastfeeding, we've seen people fight the powers that be and win.

Patty learned firsthand the challenges associated with being a professional while breastfeeding when she was studying to become a family nurse practitioner. She had recently had her fourth child, Levon. Because Levon was young and Patty knew the importance of breastfeeding, she took him to class with her. Early on, her professors tried to keep her from doing this. She argued that this was a particularly ridiculous policy for a nursing program, as nursing more than any other branch of medicine is dedicated to compassion and caring, and at that time her program included an abundance of current or expectant young mothers. In addition, her professors knew full well the importance of breastfeeding for an infant.

In response to Patty's kickback against this policy, the administration backed down and she was allowed to take her baby to class with her as long as he didn't disturb other students, a reasonable and important condition.

Later, during her graduation ceremony, Levon was with Dr. O and their other children in the audience. As the ceremony wore on, he started to cry; it was clear he wanted his mother. Neither his older siblings nor his father could comfort him, so instead of leaving and missing the ceremony, Dr. O brought him to Patty.

A few minutes later when her name was called, she stood with her baby in her arms and received a huge ovation. As she approached the stage, she realized it made sense for Levon to be there; after all, he had taken all the classes!

To end this chapter on breastfeeding, we'd like to add a few of our thoughts on pregnancy. Pregnancy, which obviously precedes breastfeeding, is not and should not be treated as a disease. The medicalization of pregnancy, birth, and breastfeeding is a controversial topic that has led to several books and films. *The Continuum Concept* by Jean Liedloff encourages holding, carrying, and breastfeeding your baby, and in the documentary film *The Business of Being Born*, actress Ricki Lake advocates a more natural approach to birth. In addition, the overuse of certain so-called routine procedures such as ultrasound in low-risk pregnancies and routine glucose tolerance tests as well as the overuse of the Doppler to obsessively listen to the baby's heartbeat should be questioned. As a Cochrane Review found, "Based on existing evidence, routine late pregnancy ultrasound in low-risk or unselected populations does not confer benefit on mother or baby."[13]

Finally, to wax philosophical for one moment, every pregnant woman is sacred and should be revered. A new chapter is being written, full of peace and turmoil, joy and pain. Remember, despite all the prodding, sticking, scoping, calculating, sterilizing, and normalizing by naive doctors, pregnancy is a uniquely powerful, even mystical event. The eternal light of life is being passed to a new generation, and past, present, and future exists as one within you. You are now more than only you. Another being carrying the hope of the future is being formed. Though empowering, pregnancy can be very tiring, so rest when you feel you need to, not when an arbitrary clock or social norm tells you to. Smile, walk in the sunshine, stare at the stars, and bathe in the moonlight. Do not worry if you don't always feel well; the threads of the natural world will guide you, as pregnancy is as natural as sleeping and waking.

Though you may have been led to believe otherwise, pregnancy and motherhood are not infirmities. On the contrary, you can do more than before, for more than just you. So embrace the moments in time that set you apart from the workaday world and experience with awe life itself. Embrace the future.

CHAPTER SIXTEEN

GET DOWN AND DIRTY

■ ■ ■

Even the most beautiful rose has been through the dirt.
—ANONYMOUS

If a healthy soil is full of death,
it is also full of life: worms, fungi, microorganisms
of all kinds. . . . Given only the health of the soil,
nothing that dies is dead for very long.
—WENDELL BERRY, *THE UNSETTLING OF AMERICA*

IN BRIEF: Avoiding all germs is a mistake. Dirt, and the rich world of microbes it contains, can be good for all of us, especially kids. There is a lot of evidence suggesting benefits from more exposure to microorganisms. Also, many hygiene products contain potentially dangerous chemicals and can irritate and dry out our skin.

According to folklore, the concept of hygiene was born thanks to the mythical Hygieia. Hygieia was the daughter of Asclepius, the Greek god of medicine. Asclepius carried a staff with a snake wrapped around it, which inspired the medical symbol still in use to this day. According to some versions of the myth, the snake would whisper the secrets of the earth in Asclepius's ear, helping him to be effective as a physician. He was so effective that he was able to cure death, a practice that angered the gods and caused Zeus to hurl a lightning bolt at him, incinerating him.

Hygieia's contribution to the healing arts was less dramatic but equally important. She would bathe and clean the sick in her father's hospitals. Her story provides evidence that the ancient Greeks recognized the importance of cleanliness in helping to restore health to the sick. But it took some time for hygiene's full significance to be realized.

For centuries humans have bathed and washed their hands regularly, but it wasn't until more recently, with the advent of germ theory, that society started to understand the extent to which disease is spread by person-to-person contact. This emerging realization led to many positive public health initiatives. In 1854, British physician John Snow realized a deadly London cholera outbreak was caused by cesspools contaminating water supplies.

Today our water supplies thankfully remain generally free of contamination and of most (but unfortunately not all) harmful chemicals, and we have many important hygiene practices that continue to prevent the spread of disease and save lives. But sometimes in our germaphobic world, with our sanitized, wash-our-hands-twice-just-to-be-sure-and-if-in-doubt-get-the-antiseptic-out culture, we are killing not only bad bacteria and germs but many good ones as well. There is a good deal of evidence all this hygiene is making us less healthy and more susceptible to allergies and autoimmune conditions. It appears that like so many other behaviors we've examined in this book, cleanliness is best when practiced in—you guessed it—moderation, along with common sense.

It turns out that dirt, and the army of invisible, often helpful bacteria that comes with it, can be good for us. According to the ironically titled hygiene hypothesis, most modern environments are too clean for children to get exposure to the variety of germs necessary for their immune system to develop properly, making them more susceptible to possible illnesses and allergies.

Allergies occur when the immune system reacts to something it may not need to react to, like the body's version of a car alarm system's going off when an innocent bystander walks nearby. Many studies have suggested that when children are exposed to more bacteria early on in life, their immune systems are better able to recognize true threats.

One of the immortal traditions of childhood is the five-second rule, which holds that if you drop food on the floor and pick it up before five seconds have passed, it's fine to eat. This rule doesn't hold scientific water, as bacteria can adhere to food as soon as it makes contact with the floor. But proponents of the hygiene hypothesis suggest it's okay for parents to allow their children to follow the natural dirt-accumulating instincts of childhood. They also say kids should play in the dirt and mud, and parents should not fight their children's propensity to lick things (all within reason, in places where there are no likely contaminants—that is to say, none of these rules apply to public bathrooms or barnyard floors or anywhere there's a good chance of coming in contact with excrement of any kind).

When we delivered babies at home in Oregon back in the 1970s, we noticed that many of our patients tried to be as sterile around the newborn as possible. They would not allow anyone but the immediate family to come near the baby right after birth. Even though these were home births, the family often would continue to wear white gowns, surgical masks, and even plastic gloves to "protect" the infant from germs long after the baby was born.

The main exception to this practice were some of the more recent immigrant families, who once the baby was born would sing, dance, and pass him or her around to what seemed like all of their family and friends. At first this practice made us nervous, to say the least, but we soon found that the babies who were kept as sterile as possible suffered from more allergies and colds than the babies who had been passed around and "exposed." We never completed an actual clinical study, but this was definitely our observation.

Today the evidence in support of this dirt- and germ-welcoming practice is compelling. A 2016 study reported in *The New England Journal of Medicine* found that Amish children who grew up close to barnyard animals had far lower rates of allergies and asthma than Hutterite children who were raised away from animals, despite the two groups having similar genetic ancestry and lifestyles.[1]

Previous studies have found a similar association between farm living and decreased incidence of asthma.[2] There's also further research suggesting that children who put their hands in their mouths are less likely to develop allergies. Researchers in New Zealand studied about 1,000 people from their birth in the 1970s until they were thirty-eight years old. They found that those who were thumb-suckers or nail-biters tended to develop common allergies less often than those who kept their hands away from their mouths most of the time. This association continued even when the researchers adjusted for confounding factors.[3]

Another study found an association between the soap used in baby wipes and an increased chance of allergies in mice, suggesting that the use of baby wipes on human babies could increase a child's chance of developing allergies.[4]

When it comes to adding more dirt—and therefore more beneficial microdiversity—to your life, dogs are a big help, as all of us who have ever had a wet dog walk through our living room know. Our four-legged friends seem to help re-create some of the conditions of farm living because of the way they track in germs—from stepping in dirt, rolling in mud, smelling excrement, and all the other charming and gross things dogs do. Having a dog around the house can raise levels of fifty-six different classes of bacteria compared with having a cat in residence, which raises only twenty-four different classes. Cats are naturally cleaner, and yes, in this instance, that is counterintuitively a bad thing.[5]

"A child growing up with a dog will have a 13 percent reduction in the likelihood of developing asthma, which seems remarkable when you remember that the majority of immunologists associated with asthma therapy regard dogs as 'causes' of the disease, or at least active exacerbations, rather than protectors," write Jack Gilbert and Rob Knight in *Dirt Is Good*. "Similarly, those growing up on a farm will have a 50 percent reduction in the likelihood of developing asthma, for many of the same reasons."

Gilbert and Knight add, "When scientists first started to tease apart the hygiene hypothesis, they found tight correlations between the likelihood of a child developing an allergy or asthma and the number of plant and animal species found within one mile of his or her home. Local biodiversity seems to play a role in mediating your child's immune experience."[6]

In addition to pet ownership, strategies for increasing your microdiversity favored by proponents of the hygiene hypothesis include gardening and not oversanitizing your house. That doesn't mean it should be dirty or dusty, but it shouldn't be like a sterile hospital operating room either. Use bleach sparingly and wash dishes by hand when you can. Cleaning dishes by hand in hot water doesn't kill as many bacteria, which sounds gross but is actually a good thing, as research indicates that people from households where dishes were handwashed have fewer allergies and less asthma than those from households where dishes were washed exclusively in the dishwasher.[7]

The health benefits of a little dirt extend to adults as well as children. In our efforts to sterilize everything in life, what we're doing is making ourselves less adaptable, less flexible, less accepting, and less healthy mentally, emotionally, and physically. Even when it comes to diet, sterile is not always best. Although stricter hygienic methods in controlling harmful bacteria is important, the natural tendency of substances like breast milk, raw milk, and raw cheese to promote a normal intestinal microbiota in humans is important for a healthy immune system.

When it comes to handwashing, the best bet, as always, is common sense. There are times when it's appropriate and other times when it is overdone. While research into exactly where and when washing hands is best is still forthcoming, Justin and Erica Sonnenburg, both microbiologists at Stanford University, share the commonsense approach that they use with their own kids in their book *The Good Gut*. "We often do not have our children wash their hands before eating if they have just been playing in our yard, petting our dog, or gardening," they write. "However, after visiting a shopping center, hospital, petting zoo, or other area that is more likely to harbor pathogens from other humans or livestock, washing hands is mandatory. We also increase the frequency of washing during cold and flu season or if we have potentially come into contact with chemical residues (e.g., pesticides)."[8]

While it's true that washing our hands can help prevent the spread of colds and other ailments, most of us can avoid using antiseptic and antibacterial wipes or gel. Even alcohol wipes, which are better, can dry out our hands and skin, as can the overuse of soap and shampoo.

Sometimes it's not hygiene that's a problem; it's what we use in pursuit of hygiene that can cause health issues. Products designed to keep us from smelling, sweating, and looking like humans can be brimming with potentially harmful ingredients. These products include shampoo, toothpaste, mouthwash, deodorant, and antiperspirant. Even something that seems as innocuous as soap may not always be our friend.

In September 2016, the U.S. Food and Drug Administration banned the sale of soap containing a number of chemicals—including triclosan and triclocarban—that have been shown to be harmful in animal studies. About 40 percent of soaps then on the market included triclosan or triclocarban, with triclocarban making its way into many bar soaps and triclosan an ingredient in many liquid soaps.

The move came after years of lobbying from public health experts who sounded the alarm after it was demonstrated that these chemicals could disrupt the reproductive system and metabolism in animals. Many feared they would have a similar effect on humans, and the widespread use of the chemicals—which the Centers for

Disease Control and Prevention found in the urine of three-quarters of Americans—also could increase bacterial resistance to antibiotics.

As expected, not everyone supported the FDA's decision. The American Cleaning Institute, an industry group, opposed the rule and released a statement, saying: "The FDA already has in its hands data that shows the safety and effectiveness of antibacterial soaps. Manufacturers are continuing their work to provide even more science and research to fill data gaps identified by the FDA."[9]

So far the FDA has not reconsidered its stance, and although triclosan and triclocarban are no longer used in soaps, they are still permitted in a wide range of products, including toothpaste, mouthwash, deodorant, laundry detergent, fabrics, toys, and even baby pacifiers.

These are not the only antibacterial chemicals causing concern. So when using cleaning products, be sure to read the labels and understand the ingredients of products you use as best as possible. Most often old-fashioned, all-natural soap and water will do the trick just fine.

The study of dirt and bacteria exposure is continuing to yield intriguing results. For instance, there is research looking at whether helminth—parasitic worm—infections can help regulate the immune system and therefore be used as a treatment for some autoimmune-like conditions, including inflammatory bowel conditions, multiple sclerosis, asthma, and atopy.

As Helena Helmby, a researcher from the London School of Hygiene and Tropical Medicine, wrote in a 2015 paper, "Without doubt there is overwhelming evidence from animal studies that helminth infections exert strong immunomodulatory activity and are able to inhibit, alter and modify other ongoing immune responses." She adds that "some promising data has been achieved using human helminth therapy but many questions remain to be investigated."[10]

If a treatment using parasites grosses you out, you may not be a fan of this next treatment: fecal transplants. A healthy colon is teeming with good bacteria, but sometimes it is killed off as a result of a poor diet, or overuse of antibiotics. Certain types of bad bacteria, like one called Clostridium difficile, or C. diff., can overpopulate the colon, causing the condition C. diff. colitis, a potentially debilitating disease that sometimes can be deadly and is infecting an increasing number of Americans.

Still classified as an experimental treatment, a fecal transplant—or bacteriotherapy, as it is known in polite society—consists of taking stool from a person with a healthy, bacteria-rich colon and placing that stool, after it has been tested for infectious disease, inside the colon of a person with colitis, most often by means of a colonoscopy. For C. diff. colitis, these treatments have a cure rate of greater than 90 percent, with no significant side effects reported to date, according to Johns Hopkins Medicine, where the treatment is offered.[11] There are also early results indicating the treatment can be effective for other autoimmune diseases, including irritable bowel syndrome, Crohn's disease, and ulcerative colitis.

Speaking of fecal matter, cleaning up with toilet paper after using the bathroom is not as hygienic or potentially healthy as using a bidet, the cleaning method favored by much of the rest of the Western world. So seize the bidet. Whenever our good friend and colleague, the late famed professor of urology and homeopathic medicine Dr. Francisco Eizayaga, would come to America to teach, he would say, "I miss three things: my beloved wife, my dear children, and my bidet . . . but in the opposite order."

Parasitic worms, bidets, and fecal matter aside, the takeaway here is that bacterial exposure, in the right instances with commonsense precautions, can be healthy. Many germs are bad, but getting rid of all of them can be even more dangerous. So don't be a germaphobe. Take steps to be less obsessed with sterile conditions. You can start by taking a hike in the woods, walking barefoot in the grass, or just playing in a park. And bring some raw milk or cheese along for a snack. In other words, get down and dirty.

CHAPTER SEVENTEEN

HAPPINESS

Pursue It

■ ■ ■

Happiness is the meaning and
the purpose of life,
the whole aim and end of human existence.

—ARISTOTLE

IN BRIEF: Happiness is not only fulfilling and fun, it's healthy; our mental outlook has a profound effect on our overall well-being. The secret to happiness remains a secret, but family, friends, and making time for what really matters are often part of the happiness equation.

When New York City journalist Norman Cousins was diagnosed with a crippling connective tissue disease, he laughed it off . . . literally. Given a 1 in 500 chance of recovery by his doctors in the 1960s, he started taking massive amounts of vitamin C and, instead of working, spent his days watching comedies. He later would write in a famous account, "I made the joyous discovery that ten minutes of genuine belly laughter had an anesthetic effect and would give me at least two hours of pain-free sleep," adding, "When the pain-killing effect of the laughter wore off, we would switch on the motion picture projector again and, not infrequently, it would lead to another pain-free interval."[1]

Cousins said that due to his self-prescribed regimen of laughter, he recovered. He lived until 1990, decades after his original diagnosis.

Happiness is not a luxury, nor should it become a casualty of our busy lives. It is one of the reasons we were born, one of the things that makes life so very worth living, and it is the root and goal of all vices.

And while happiness is a reward in and of itself, as Cousins's case reminds us, sometimes it can help us in surprising ways and really be the best medicine. Regardless of what some skeptics say, the idea that positive thinking plays a central role in health has been shown time and again.

We turn not older with years, but newer every day.

—EMILY DICKINSON

Ellen Langer, a Harvard psychologist, has made a career of studying the mind's influence on health. In the 1980s, she recruited eight men in their seventies and had them live in an apartment in New Hampshire that had been retrofitted as a time capsule, with music, movies, TV shows, books, and magazines from 1959, when the men in the study were in their prime. There were no mirrors in the dwelling and the men were told to make an attempt to be the person they were twenty-two years before. They were told that if they did that, they would feel as they used to.

The results, which were staggering, included improvements in dexterity, agility, posture, and eyesight. This wasn't the first or last time Langer's work produced spectacular results. Previously she had found that nursing home residents who were in the early stages of memory loss did better on memory tests when they were given incentives for remembering. In another classic study, she gave plants to different groups of nursing home residents. One group had to take care of the plants themselves; the other group had the plants taken care of by the staff. A year and a half later, twice as many residents who took care of their plants themselves were alive than those whose plants were taken care of for them.

More recently, Langer and a student, Alia Crum, studied eighty-four hotel chambermaids who reported they did not exercise much. One group was told how much exercise they actually got while cleaning rooms, and it was explained to them that this was as much, and possibly more, exercise than the surgeon general recommends. Once their mind-set had been changed, the maids lost more weight relative to a control group who had not been given a new perspective about the exercise inherent in their work.[2]

In 2010, Langer was a coauthor of a study at a hair salon where women were given blood pressure tests before and after a haircut and or a hair-coloring appointment. Participants said they felt they looked younger after the makeover, and they also had lower blood pressure.[3]

In Bruce Grierson's 2014 *New York Times Magazine* article about Langer, Jeffrey Rediger, a psychiatrist, said of her: "She's one of the people at Harvard who really get it. . . . That health and illness are much more rooted in our minds and in our hearts and how we experience ourselves in the world than our models even begin to understand." Much of her work examines people's perception of the world around them and their need to focus attention on what is right in front of them. In other words, their need to be there.[4]

Research into the ways positive thinking helps our health still is ongoing, but it's also clear that the opposite is true: negative thinking can have a dramatic effect on us. Extreme grief even can precipitate death from a "broken heart," which, although it may sound made up, is a real thing. According to the American Heart Association, "Broken heart syndrome, also called stress-induced cardiomyopathy or takotsubo cardiomyopathy, can strike even if you're healthy." Some potential emotional shocks that can precipitate broken heart syndrome include the death of a loved one, bad news including a negative medical diagnosis, losing (or winning) at a casino, the loss of a job, or the breakup of a marriage, as well as physical shocks including accidents, major surgery, or even some drugs.[5]

When actress Debbie Reynolds died in 2016, just a day after the death of her equally famous daughter Carrie Fisher, some speculated a broken heart was the cause. Though that turned out not to be the case (Reynolds died of a stroke), her son, Todd Fisher, said grief was a factor.

Find ecstasy in life; the mere sense of living is joy enough.

—EMILY DICKINSON

Though the mind-body connection is not fully understood, and serious study of the issue has sometimes been hijacked by the "wellness" industry and its clever marketing slogans, the connection between what we think and what we feel is real. Which brings us to the obvious next question: How do we obtain happiness?

If we knew that, we'd be doing more than just writing this book, but we can tell you many of those who have studied happiness conclude that the things we think will make us happy—winning the lottery, a big promotion at work, etc.—often provide less of an uptick in joy than we expect. Lasting happiness doesn't come just from what we drink, eat, or do—not even the great things we've talked about drinking, eating, and doing elsewhere in this book. Instead, it comes from the people with whom we do all those things and the kindness we share. Family and friends can make us crazy sometimes, but they also offer the keys to contentment.

Passing stranger! You do not know how longingly I look upon you,
You must be he I was seeking, or she I was seeking,
(it comes to me, as of a dream,)
I have somewhere surely lived a life of joy with you.

—WALT WHITMAN

According to research presented at the 125th annual convention of the American Psychological Association in 2017, loneliness and social isolation present a greater public health hazard than obesity. Those with stronger social connections had a 50 percent decreased chance of death, while the impact from the isolation and loneliness epidemic continues to grow.

"Being connected to others socially is widely considered a fundamental human need—crucial to both well-being and survival. Extreme examples show infants in custodial care who lack human contact fail to thrive and often die and, indeed, social isolation or solitary confinement has been used as a form of punishment," Julianne Holt-Lunstad, Ph.D., a professor of psychology at Brigham Young University, said when the research was presented. "Yet an increasing portion of the U.S. population now experiences isolation regularly."

About 42.6 million people over age forty-five in the United States are estimated to be suffering from chronic loneliness, according to AARP's 2010 Loneliness Study. And the picture gets more solitary from there: Most recent U.S. census data showed more than a quarter of the population lives alone, more than half of the population is unmarried, and marriage rates and the number of children per household have declined.[6]

In 2009, George Vaillant, the longest-serving former director of one of the most comprehensive longitudinal studies on healthy male adults, the Harvard Study of Adult Development (previously known as the Grant Study in Social Adjustments), was asked by *The Atlantic* what he thought was the most important finding of the study, started in the 1930s. He replied, "The only thing that really matters in life are your relations to other people."[7]

As if a phantom caress'd me, I thought I was not alone,
walking here by the shore;
But the one I thought was with me, as now I walk by the shore—
the one I loved, that caress'd me,
As I lean and look through the glimmering light—
that one has utterly disappear'd,
And those appear that are hateful to me, and mock me.

—WALT WHITMAN

So visit or call your mother, daughter, sibling, or grandparent and take a walk together. Or simply take a hike with your four-footed best friend, gaze in awe at the horizon, relax your eyes, rest your mind, and savor the moment in nature. Make new connections with those in your community by joining a volunteer, exercise, or spiritual group, or by signing up for a class. Or best of all, hug somebody. A hug a day really can keep the doctor away. In a 2015 study involving 404 healthy adults, researchers from Carnegie Mellon University examined the effects of social support and hugs on the susceptibility of developing the common cold after being exposed to the virus. Those who got more support and hugs were less likely to get a cold, or if they did develop a cold were more likely to have milder symptoms.[8]

But what about connections made via technology, through smartphones, the Internet, and social networks? These are more complicated.

In a 1998 study, Robert E. Kraut, a researcher at Carnegie Mellon University, found the more that participants used the

Internet, the more their depression increased. More recently, Kraut says that has changed. When his 1998 study was conducted in the early days of the Internet, people were communicating with people they did not know across the globe, what Kraut calls "weak ties." As Adam Piore writes in *Nautilus*, "Kraut's more recent research has found that today most people spend their time online communicating with people with whom they already have strong ties. In those cases, he argues, the findings are unequivocal: Online connection decreases depression, reduces loneliness, and increases levels of perceived social support."[9]

But as anyone who has gone out with friends or family who were constantly looking at their smartphones knows, technology can be a double-edged sword when it comes to real connections. In addition to robbing us of actual face time with those physically near us in the real world, technology can rob us of an essential element of happiness and a modern vice that is increasingly difficult to come by: free time.

In a 2016 report, an app tracked the cell phone habits of more than ninety smartphone users. They found people tapped, swiped, and clicked on their phones an average of 2,617 times a day.[10] While some of these "touches" are no doubt responses to work emails, important texts, and even trivial but harmless fun updates, it seems likely that smartphone use is also an addictive habit. Like so much else we discuss in this book, the key is moderation. Computers, phones, and technology in general can be useful—while writing this book we emailed, texted, and collaborated in real time with digital documents. This is one example of the many ways we find technology helpful in our daily lives, but we always try to make sure we are the ones using the technology, not the other way around.

Phones also can increase our FOMO (fear of missing out) and lead us to clutter our lives with busy but unrewarding activities as we attempt to keep up with the Joneses, or at least the upbeat way the Joneses portray themselves online.

Of all the things that matter in life—friends, family, good food, good entertainment, fresh air, fresh water—very little of that has been improved by technology. Ultimately, the things that always have mattered to humans still matter: the quality of how we conduct and share our lives with people around us and with nature.

Even potentially good things, like school and work, can be thieves of time.

The satirical paper and website *The Onion* once ran the headline: "Health Experts Recommend Standing Up at Desk, Leaving Office, Never Coming Back." "We observed significant physical and mental health benefits in subjects after just one instance of standing up, walking out the door, and never coming back to their place of work again," said the made-up authors of the fictional study. "We encourage Americans to experiment with stretching their legs by strolling across their office and leaving all their responsibilities behind forever just one time to see how much better they feel. People tend to become more productive, motivated, and happy almost immediately."[11]

This tongue-in-cheek article is not as far off as you might think.

Americans are retiring later, and the health of the elderly is declining. As *The Boston Globe* reported in October 2017, new data suggests that "Americans' health is declining and millions of middle-age workers face the prospect of shorter, and less active, retirements than their parents enjoyed."[12]

School or work, despite their obvious benefits, can sometimes be unhealthy. Sitting for eight uninterrupted hours a day in a windowless office or classroom isn't good for us; neither is the eyestrain caused by constant reading, often on electronic screens. Spending so much of our lives indoors being sedentary can diminish our mental, emotional, and physical health.

None of what's been discussed in this chapter means we shouldn't grieve the loss of loved ones or avoid all stress in search of a blissful, blemish-free life. Happiness, like the other vices in this book, is best when enjoyed in moderation. It's okay to be sad, it's okay to be angry, but when our defense mechanism, or vital force, is working well, we should not get stuck in never-ending cycles of sadness, anxiety, fear, or anger. And when you do get sad or angry, allow yourself that sadness. In other words, don't worry too much about not being happy, and don't despair if you're not presently jumping for joy. While many studies have found a link between positive and happy feelings and health, one large study of more than a million middle-aged women in the UK found no increased chance of death for less happy women over a ten-year period.[13]

The nice thing about fun is even when it's not helping us healthwise, it's certainly helping our mental state because it's, you know, fun. Elsewhere in this book we've talked about many vices that we and others enjoy. To maximize your enjoyment, we recommend looking forward to one or more each day and really savoring that joyful experience, paying attention while you're engaging in it, and telling others about it. In a nutshell, try to live *la dolce vita*, "the sweet life." The book *Living La Dolce Vita: Bring the Passion, Laughter, and Serenity of Italy into Your Daily Life* by Raeleen D'Agostino Mautner celebrates some of the most important aspects of the sweet life. These include making the simple decision to prepare and share healthy delicious food and drink with friends and family in a fun, loving, positive, and open environment.[14]

So limit stress, but don't avoid it entirely. Take heart in the words of the poet Henry Wadsworth Longfellow:

> *Not enjoyment, and not sorrow,*
> *Is our destined end or way;*
> *But to act, that each to-morrow*
> *Find us farther than to-day.*

If you forget everything else about this book, remember these four words: Don't worry, be happy.

AFTERWORD

In August 2017, the oldest man then alive, Israel Kristal, died. He was a month shy of his 114th birthday.

A Jewish native of Poland, he had survived the Holocaust and was recognized as the world's oldest man by Guinness World Records the previous year. Unable to celebrate his bar mitzvah when he turned thirteen because of World War I, he celebrated it a hundred years later at the age of 113.

When reporters asked him for health advice, he was reluctant to offer any. "There have been smarter, stronger, and better-looking men than me who are no longer alive. All that is left for us to do is to keep on working as hard as we can and rebuild what is lost," he said.

We understand his reluctance.

Born in 1903, Kristal had seen the beliefs of people and nations shift and change. He lived through two world wars and saw humans walk on the moon, harness the energy of an atom, peer at subatomic particles, map the human genome, and develop theories of time and space. At the time when he was born, people ate unprocessed food, babies breastfed, and it was considered okay to eat things like fat and drink some beer. Later that all changed, but now in some ways the pendulum is shifting back toward the way things were.

As we've noted elsewhere in this book, health and science are always changing. What we believe might be true today may not be true in the future. Our examination of the "good vices" in this book is based on studies and our personal experiences, and is meant to entertain and inspire further thought and research.

We believe that having fun and being healthy do not have to be mutually exclusive pursuits, and that an enjoyable and healthy diet and lifestyle are often one and the same. The specifics of which vices might be good ones have changed in the past and almost certainly will change again in the future. When practicing your own good vices, remember to follow common sense and not to be overly swayed by the latest news-grabbing headline, whether good or bad. Always share the fun with those you love and those you meet along the way.

In the end, much of medicine relies on current science and some guesswork, and our best guess is that doing something that you enjoy and that makes you happy—in moderation and within reason—is healthier than people think. But that's just a guess.

As Kristal humbly told the Guinness officials after 113 years of observing this world: "I don't know the secret for long life. I believe that everything is determined from above and we shall never know the reasons why."[1]

ACKNOWLEDGMENTS

Special thanks and deepest gratitude to Ann Godoff of Penguin Press for her encouragement, support, advice, and immeasurable kindness.

Thanks to Sara Carder, Joanna Ng, and the whole Tarcher-Perigee team.

Thanks to Lyn Hottes and Josh Pahigian for their help and writing guidance.

Thanks to Chris for keeping us all in line. One love.

SUGGESTED READING

Airola, Paavo, Ph.D. *How to Get Well*. Sherwood, OR: Health Plus Publishers, 1984.

Bates, William. *The Bates Method for Better Eyesight Without Glasses*, revised edition. New York: Henry Holt, 1981.

Bieler, Henry G., M.D. *Food Is Your Best Medicine*. New York: Ballantine Books, 1990.

Buettner, Dan. *The Blue Zones: Nine Lessons for Living Longer from the People Who've Lived the Longest*, second edition. Washington, D.C.: National Geographic Society, 2012.

Cummings, Stephen, M.D., and Dana Ullman. *Everybody's Guide to Homeopathic Medicines*, revised edition. New York: Tarcher, 2004.

Fallon, Sally. *Nourishing Traditions: The Cookbook That Challenges Politically Correct Nutrition and Diet Dictocrats*, second revised edition. Washington, D.C.: NewTrends Publishing, 2001.

Gaskin, Ina May. *Spiritual Midwifery*, fourth edition. Summertown, TN: Book Publishing Company, 2004.

Gilbert, Jack, and Rob Knight. *Dirt Is Good: The Advantage of Germs for Your Child's Developing Immune System*. New York: St. Martin's Press, 2017.

Hahnemann, Samuel. *The Organon of Medicine*, fifth and sixth editions. Gazelle Distribution Trade, 2009.

Hazan, Marcella. *The Essentials of Classic Italian Cooking*. New York: Knopf, 1992.

Kirsch, Irving. *The Emperor's New Drugs: Exploding the Antidepressant Myth*. New York: Basic Books, 2010.

Suggested Reading

La Leche League International. *The Womanly Art of Breastfeeding*, eighth revised edition. New York: Ballantine Books, 2010.

Liedloff, Jean. *The Continuum Concept*. Perseus Books, 1977.

Lindlahr, Henry. *Nature Cure: Philosophy and Practice Based on the Unity of Disease and Cure*. Nature Cure Publishing Company, 1917.

Ofgang, Erik. *Buzzed: Beers, Booze, and Coffee Brews—Where to Find the Best Craft Beverages in New England*. Yarmouth, ME: Islandport Press, 2016.

Oster, Emily. *Expecting Better: Why the Conventional Pregnancy Wisdom Is Wrong and What You Really Need to Know*, revised edition. New York: Penguin Press, 2016.

Panos, Maesimund B., M.D., and Jane Heimlich. *Homeopathic Medicine at Home*. New York: Tarcher, 1980.

Pizzorno, Joseph E. *Textbook of Natural Medicine*, fourth edition. Churchill Livingstone, 2012.

Pollan, Michael. *In Defense of Food: An Eater's Manifesto*. New York: Penguin Press, 2008.

Price, Weston A., DDS. *Nutrition and Physical Degeneration*, eighth edition. Lemon Grove, CA: Price-Pottenger Nutrition Foundation, 2009.

Sonnenburg, Justin, and Erica Sonnenburg. *The Good Gut*. New York: Penguin Press, 2015.

Ullman, Dana. *Homeopathic Medicine for Children and Infants*. New York: Tarcher, 1992.

Vithoulkas, George. *Homeopathy: Medicine of the New Man*. New York: Touchstone, 1979.

NOTES

INTRODUCTION

1. Martin A. Makary and Michael Daniel. "Medical Error—The Third Leading Cause of Death in the U.S." *BMJ: British Medical Journal* 353 (2016): i2139.

2. Dima Mazen Qato, Katharine Ozenberger, and Mark Olfson. "Prevalence of Prescription Medications with Depression as a Potential Adverse Effect Among Adults in the United States." *JAMA* 319.22 (2018): 2289–98.

3. John Crewdson. "Statistics Misleading, Some Doctors Say." *Chicago Tribune,* March 15, 2002; http://articles.chicagotribune.com/2002-03-15 /news/0203150271_1_mammography-breast-cancer-death-benefit. Accessed September 21, 2017.

4. Robert E. Kelly et al. "Relationship Between Drug Company Funding and Outcomes of Clinical Psychiatric Research." *Psychological Medicine* 36.11 (2006): 1647–56.

5. Bernard Lo and Marilyn J. Field, eds. *Conflict of Interest in Medical Research, Education, and Practice.* Washington, D.C.: National Academies Press, 2009.

6. P. C. Gøtzsche and K. Jørgensen. "Screening for Breast Cancer with Mammography." Cochrane, June 4, 2013; https://www.cochrane.org/CD001877 /BREASTCA_screening-for-breast-cancer-with-mammography. Accessed July 24, 2018.

7. Karsten Juhl Jørgensen et al. "Breast Cancer Screening in Denmark: A Cohort Study of Tumor Size and Overdiagnosis." *Annals of Internal Medicine* 166.5 (2017): 313–23.

8. Matthew P. Lungren et al. "Physician Self-Referral: Frequency of Negative Findings at MR Imaging of the Knee as a Marker of Appropriate Utilization." *Radiology* 269.3 (2013): 810–15.

9. J. Bruce Moseley et al. "A Controlled Trial of Arthroscopic Surgery for Osteoarthritis of the Knee." *New England Journal of Medicine* 347 (2002): 81–88; "A Fascinating Landmark Study of Placebo Surgery for Knee Osteoarthritis." November 10, 2016; https://www.painscience.com/biblio/fascinating-landmark-study-of-placebo-surgery-for-knee-osteoarthritis.html. Accessed October 3, 2017.

10. Centers for Disease Control and Prevention. "CDC: 1 in 3 Antibiotic Prescriptions Unnecessary." May 3, 2016; https://www.cdc.gov/media/releases/2016/p0503-unnecessary-prescriptions.html. Accessed September 30, 2017.

11. Irving Kirsch. "Antidepressants and the Placebo Effect." *Zeitschrift für Psychologie* 222.3 (2014): 128–34.

12. Peter C. Gøtzsche. "Antidepressants Increase the Risk of Suicide, Violence, and Homicide at All Ages." *BMJ* 358 (2017): j36n7; https://www.bmj.com/content/358/bmj.j3697/rr-4. Accessed June 10, 2018.

13. "VBAC Birth: Success Rates, Risks, and How to Prepare." Mama Natural; https://www.mamanatural.com/vbac/. Accessed October 7, 2017.

CHAPTER 1. A BEER A DAY JUST MIGHT HELP KEEP THE DOCTOR AWAY

1. "Alcohol: Balancing Risks and Benefits." The Nutrition Source, Harvard T. H. Chan School of Public Health; https://www.hsph.harvard.edu/nutritionsource/alcohol-full-story/. Accessed February 10, 2017.

2. Centers for Disease Control and Prevention. "Frequently Asked Questions: Alcohol and Public Health," October 18, 2016; https://www.cdc.gov/alcohol/faqs.htm. Accessed February 11, 2017.

3. "Beer Compound Shows Potent Promise in Prostate Cancer Battle." Oregon State University Newsroom, September 30, 2009; https://today.oregonstate

Notes

.edu/archives/2006/may/beer-compound-shows-potent-promise-prostate
-cancer-battle. Accessed June 24, 2017.

4. "Compound from Hops Aids Cognitive Function in Young Animals." Oregon State University Newsroom, September 22, 2014; https://today.oregonstate .edu/archives/2014/sep/compound-hops-aids-cognitive-function-young -animals. Accessed June 24, 2017.

5. "Hops Extract Studied to Prevent Breast Cancer." Science Daily, July 11, 2016; https://www.sciencedaily.com/releases/2016/07/160711151705.htm. Accessed June 24, 2017.

6. Paolo Boffetta and Lawrence Garfinkel. "Alcohol Drinking and Mortality Among Men Enrolled in an American Cancer Society Prospective Study." *Epidemiology* 1.5 (1990): 342–48.

7. Morten Grønbaek et al. "Changes in Alcohol Intake and Mortality: A Longitudinal Population-Based Study." *Epidemiology* 15.2 (2004): 222–28.

8. Annie Britton, Archana Singh-Manoux, and Michael Marmot. "Alcohol Consumption and Cognitive Function in the Whitehall II Study." *American Journal of Epidemiology* 160.3 (2004): 240–47.

9. Marge Dwyer. "Moderate Alcohol Intake May Decrease Men's Risk for Type 2 Diabetes." Harvard T. H. Chan School of Public Health, February 15, 2011; https://www.hsph.harvard.edu/news/features/moderate-alcohol-intake-may -decrease-mens-risk-for-type-2-diabetes/. Accessed February 11, 2017.

10. David Stauth. "Anti-Cancer Compound in Beer Gaining Interest." Oregon State University Newsroom, October 25, 2005; https://today.oregonstate .edu/archives/2005/oct/anti-cancer-compound-beer-gaining-interest. Accessed February 11, 2017.

11. David Stauth. "Xanthohumol in Lab Tests Lowers Cholesterol, Blood Sugar, and Weight Gain." Oregon State University, April 18, 2016; https: //today.oregonstate.edu/archives/2016/apr/xanthohumol-lab-tests-lowers -cholesterol-blood-sugar-and-weight-gain. Accessed February 11, 2017.

12. Simona Costanzo et al. "Wine, Beer or Spirit Drinking in Relation to Fatal and Non-Fatal Cardiovascular Events: A Meta-Analysis." *European Journal of Epidemiology* 26.11 (2011): 833–50.

13. Chiara Scoccianti et al. "Female Breast Cancer and Alcohol Consumption: A Review of the Literature." *American Journal of Preventive Medicine* 46.3, Suppl. 1 (2014): S16–S25.

14. Shumin Zhang et al. "A Prospective Study of Folate Intake and the Risk of Breast Cancer." *JAMA* 281.17 (1999): 1632–37.

15. Max G. Griswold et al. "Alcohol Use and Burden for 195 Countries and Territories, 1990–2016: A Systematic Analysis for the Global Burden of Disease Study 2016." *The Lancet* 392.10152 (2018): P1015–P1035.

16. David Spiegelhalter. "The Risks of Alcohol (Again)." Winton Centre for Risk and Evidence Communication, August 23, 2018; https://medium .com/wintoncentre/the-risks-of-alcohol-again-2ae8cb006a4a. Accessed September 13, 2018.

17. "Alcohol: Balancing Risks and Benefits." The Nutrition Source, Harvard T. H. Chan School of Public Health; https://www.hsph.harvard.edu /nutritionsource/alcohol-full-story/. Accessed February 12, 2017.

CHAPTER 2. WINE, WINE, SO VERY FINE

1. "Alcohol: Balancing Risks and Benefits." The Nutrition Source, Harvard T. H. Chan School of Public Health; https://www.hsph.harvard.edu /nutritionsource/alcohol-full-story/. Accessed February 10, 2017.

2. Yftach Gepner et al. "Effects of Initiating Moderate Alcohol Intake on Cardiometabolic Risk in Adults with Type 2 Diabetes, a 2-Year Random- ized, Controlled Trial." *Annals of Internal Medicine* 163.8 (2015): 569–79.

3. Joseph C. Anderson et al. "Prevalence and Risk of Colorectal Neoplasia in Consumers of Alcohol in a Screening Population." *American Journal of Gastroenterology* 100.9 (2005): 2049–55.

4. Marge Dwyer. "Moderate Alcohol Intake May Decrease Men's Risk for Type 2 Diabetes." Harvard T. H. Chan School of Public Health News, February 15, 2011, https://www.hsph.harvard.edu/news/features/moderate-alcohol -intake-may-decrease-mens-risk-for-type-2-diabetes/. Accessed February 11, 2017.

5. Sonia Navarro et al. "Inhaled Resveratrol Treatments Slow Ageing-Related Degenerative Changes in Mouse Lung." *Thorax* 72.5 (2017): thoraxjnl-2016.

6. Joseph A. Baur et al. "Resveratrol Improves Health and Survival of Mice on a High-Calorie Diet." *Nature* 444.7117 (2006): 337–42.

7. R. Corder et al. "Oenology: Red Wine Procyanidins and Vascular Health." *Nature* 444.7119 (2006): 566.

8. Timo E. Strandberg et al. "Alcoholic Beverage Preference, 29-Year Mortality, and Quality of Life in Men in Old Age." *The Journals of Gerontology Series A: Biological Sciences and Medical Sciences* 62.2 (2007): 213–18.

CHAPTER 3. MOVED BY THE SPIRITS

1. "Alcohol: Balancing Risks and Benefits." The Nutrition Source, Harvard T. H. Chan School of Public Health; https://www.hsph.harvard.edu /nutritionsource/alcohol-full-story/. Accessed November 18, 2017.

2. Trevor Thompson et al. "Analgesic Effects of Alcohol: A Systematic Review and Meta-Analysis of Controlled Experimental Studies in Healthy Participants." *Journal of Pain* 18.5 (2017): 499–510.

3. Andrew F. Jarosz, Gregory J. H. Colflesh, and Jennifer Wiley. "Uncorking the Muse: Alcohol Intoxication Facilitates Creative Problem Solving." *Consciousness and Cognition* 21.1 (2012): 487–93. Benjamin C. Storm and Trisha N. Patel. "Forgetting as a Consequence and Enabler of Creative Thinking." *Journal of Experimental Psychology: Learning, Memory, and Cognition* 40.6 (2014): 1594–1609.

4. Kew-Kim Chew et al. "Alcohol Consumption and Male Erectile Dysfunction: An Unfounded Reputation for Risk?" *Journal of Sexual Medicine* 6.5 (2009): 1386–94.

CHAPTER 4. SLEEP: LIFE'S MEDITATION

1. Sirimon Reutrakul and Eve Van Cauter. "Interactions Between Sleep, Circadian Function, and Glucose Metabolism: Implications for Risk and

Severity of Diabetes." *Annals of the New York Academy of Sciences* 1311.1 (2014): 151–73.

2. Centers for Disease Control and Prevention. "Sleep and Sleep Disorders— Sleep and Chronic Disease." July 1, 2013; http://www.cdc.gov/sleep /about_sleep/chronic_disease.html. Accessed June 10, 2017.

3. "Researchers Are Studying the Link Between Sleep and Cancer." Cancer Treatment Centers of America; https://thecancerspecialist.com/2018/04/10 /researchers-are-studying-the-link-between-sleep-and-cancer/. Accessed June 10, 2017.

4. Sanjay R. Patel et al. "Association Between Reduced Sleep and Weight Gain in Women." *American Journal of Epidemiology* 164.10 (2006): 947–54.

5. Sanjay R. Patel and Frank B. Hu. "Short Sleep Duration and Weight Gain: A Systematic Review." *Obesity* 16.3 (2008): 643–53.

6. Earl S. Ford, Timothy J. Cunningham, and Janet B. Croft. "Trends in Self-Reported Sleep Duration Among U.S. Adults from 1985 to 2012." *Sleep* 38.5 (2015): 829–32.

7. Ullrich Wagner et al. "Sleep Inspires Insight." *Nature* 427.6972 (2004): 352–55.

8. Sara C. Mednick et al. "The Restorative Effect of Naps on Perceptual Deterioration." *Nature Neuroscience* 5.7 (2002): 677.

9. Kyla L. Wahlstrom et al. "Examining the Impact of Later School Start Times on the Health and Academic Performance of High School Students: A Multi-Site Study." Center for Applied Research and Educational Improvement. St. Paul: University of Minnesota, 2014.

10. "Let Them Sleep: AAP Recommends Delaying Start Times of Middle and High Schools to Combat Teen Sleep Deprivation." American Academy of Pediatrics, August 25, 2014; https://www.aap.org/en-us/about-the-aap/aap -press-room/pages/let-them-sleep-aap-recommends-delaying-start -times-of-middle-and-high-schools-to-combat-teen-sleep-deprivation.aspx. Accessed June 10, 2017.

11. "AMA Supports Delayed School Start Times to Improve Adolescent Well-

ness." American Medical Association, June 14, 2016; https://www.ama-assn.org/ama-supports-delayed-school-start-times-improve-adolescent-wellness. Accessed June 10, 2017.

12. Charlotte Graham-McLay. "A 4-Day Workweek? A Test Run Shows a Surprising Result." *New York Times*, July 19, 2018; https://www.nytimes.com/2018/07/19/world/asia/four-day-workweek-new-zealand.html. Accessed July 22, 2018.

13. Ben Carter et al. "Association Between Portable Screen-Based Media Device Access or Use and Sleep Outcomes: A Systematic Review and Meta-Analysis." *JAMA Pediatrics* 170.12 (2016): 1202–208.

14. Mohamed Boubekri et al. "Impact of Windows and Daylight Exposure on Overall Health and Sleep Quality of Office Workers: A Case-Control Pilot Study." *Journal of Clinical Sleep Medicine* 10.6 (2014): 603–11.

CHAPTER 5. SEX, DRUGS, AND ROCK AND ROLL (OKAY, JUST SEX)

1. Josephine Brouard. "7 Unexpected Health Benefits You Get from Sex." *Reader's Digest, ND;* https://www.rd.com/advice/relationships/7-unexpected-health-benefits-you-get-from-sex/. Accessed November 11, 2017.

2. Susan A. Hall et al. "Sexual Activity, Erectile Dysfunction, and Incident Cardiovascular Events." *American Journal of Cardiology* 105.2 (2010): 192–97.

3. George Davey Smith, Stephen Frankel, and John Yarnell. "Sex and Death: Are They Related? Findings from the Caerphilly Cohort Study." *BMJ* 315.7123 (1997): 1641–44.

4. Stuart Brody. "Blood Pressure Reactivity to Stress Is Better for People Who Recently Had Penile-Vaginal Intercourse Than for People Who Had Other or No Sexual Activity." *Biological Psychology* 71.2 (2006): 214–22.

5. Julie Frappier et al. "Energy Expenditure During Sexual Activity in Young Healthy Couples." *PLOS One* 8.10 (2013): e79342.

6. Carl J. Charnetski and Francis X. Brennan. "Sexual Frequency and Salivary Immunoglobulin A (IgA)." *Psychological Reports* 94.3 (2004): 839–44.

7. Anke Hambach et al. "The Impact of Sexual Activity on Idiopathic Headaches: An Observational Study." *Cephalalgia* 33.6 (2013): 384–89.

8. David G. Blanchflower and Andrew J. Oswald. "Money, Sex and Happiness: An Empirical Study." *Scandinavian Journal of Economics* 106.3 (2004): 393–415.

9. Daniel Kahneman et al. "Toward National Well-Being Accounts." *American Economic Review* 94.2 (2004): 429–34.

10. George Loewenstein et al. "Does Increased Sexual Frequency Enhance Happiness?" *Journal of Economic Behavior & Organization* 116 (2015): 206–18.

11. Andrea Downey. "Being Single Could Kill: Scientists Discover Lonely People Are '50% More Likely to Die Young.'" *The Sun* (UK), August 7, 2017; https://www.thesun.co.uk/living/4188309/being-single-could-kill-lonely-people-50-more-likely-to-die-young/. Accessed September 16, 2017.

12. "So Lonely I Could Die." American Psychological Association, August 5, 2017; http://www.apa.org/news/press/releases/2017/08/lonely-die.aspx. Accessed September 16, 2017.

13. "Marriage and Men's Health." *Harvard Men's Health Watch*, July 1, 2010; https://www.health.harvard.edu/newsletter_article/marriage-and-mens-health. Accessed September 21, 2017.

CHAPTER 6. COFFEE: HUG A MUG

1. Ming Ding et al. "Long-Term Coffee Consumption and Risk of Cardiovascular Disease: A Systematic Review and a Dose-Response Meta-Analysis of Prospective Cohort Studies." *Circulation* 129.6 (2014): 643–59.

2. Susanna C. Larsson and Nicola Orsini. "Coffee Consumption and Risk of Stroke: A Dose-Response Meta-Analysis of Prospective Studies." *American Journal of Epidemiology* 174.9 (2011): 993–1001.

3. Chang-Hae Park et al. "Coffee Consumption and Risk of Prostate Cancer:

A Meta-Analysis of Epidemiological Studies." *BJU International* 106.6 (2010): 762–69.

4. Susanna C. Larsson and Alicja Wolk. "Coffee Consumption and Risk of Liver Cancer: A Meta-Analysis." *Gastroenterology* 132.5 (2007): 1740–45.

5. Marc J. Gunter et al. "Coffee Drinking and Mortality in 10 European Countries: A Multinational Cohort Study." *Annals of Internal Medicine* 167.4 (2017): 236–47.

6. Jacob Schor. "Coffee and Hypertension." *Natural Medicine Journal* 9.5 (2017); https://www.naturalmedicinejournal.com/journal/2017-05/coffee -and-hypertension. Accessed November 5, 2017.

7. "IARC Monographs Evaluate Drinking Coffee, Maté, and Very Hot Beverages." International Agency for Research on Cancer, World Health Organization, June 15, 2016; https://www.iarc.fr/en/media-centre /pr/2016/pdfs/pr244_E.pdf. Accessed November 5, 2017.

CHAPTER 7. CHOCOLATE: LOVE WITHOUT WORDS

1. Chun Shing Kwok et al. "Habitual Chocolate Consumption and Risk of Cardiovascular Disease Among Healthy Men and Women." *Heart* 101.16 (2015): 1279–87.

2. Susanna C. Larsson et al. "Chocolate Consumption and Risk of Myocardial Infarction: A Prospective Study and Meta-Analysis." *Heart* 102 (2016): 1017–22.

3. Brian Buijsse et al. "Chocolate Consumption in Relation to Blood Pressure and Risk of Cardiovascular Disease in German Adults." *European Heart Journal* 31.13 (2010): 1616–23.

4. Alfonso Moreira et al. "Chocolate Consumption Is Associated with a Lower Risk of Cognitive Decline." *Journal of Alzheimer's Disease* 53.1 (2016): 85–93.

5. "Dietary Flavanols Reverse Age-Related Memory Decline." Columbia University Irving Medical Center, October 26, 2014; http://newsroom

.cumc.columbia.edu/blog/2014/10/26/flavanols-memory-decline/. Accessed March 11, 2017.

6. Stephen J. Crozier et al. "Cacao Seeds Are a 'Super Fruit': A Comparative Analysis of Various Fruit Powders and Products." *Chemistry Central Journal* 5 (2011): 5. Accessed May 2, 2017.

7. Rafael Franco, Ainhoa Oñatibia-Astibia, and Eva Martínez-Pinilla. "Health Benefits of Methylxanthines in Cacao and Chocolate." *Nutrients* 5.10 (2013): 4159–73.

CHAPTER 8. SWEET-TOOTH BONANZA: HONEY, MAPLE SYRUP, AND SUGARCANE

1. Emmanouil Apostolidis et al. "In Vitro Evaluation of Phenolic-Enriched Maple Syrup Extracts for Inhibition of Carbohydrate Hydrolyzing Enzymes Relevant to Type 2 Diabetes Management." *Journal of Functional Foods* 3.2 (2011): 100–106; "Maple Syrup's Health Benefits—Unique Antioxidants." Health Impact News, September 29, 2018, http://healthimpactnews.com/2013/maple-syrups-health-benefits-unique-antioxidants/. Accessed May 21, 2017.

2. Natalie O'Neill. "Maple Syrup Isn't Just Delicious, It Also Could Cure Alzheimer's Disease." *New York Post,* March 14, 2016; http://nypost.com/2016/03/14/maple-syrup-isnt-just-delicious-it-also-could-cure-alzheimers-disease/. Accessed May 21, 2017.

3. Tricia M. Nemoseck et al. "Honey Promotes Lower Weight Gain, Adiposity, and Triglycerides Than Sucrose in Rats." *Nutrition Research* 31.1 (2011): 55–60.

4. D. Enette Larson-Meyer et al. "Effect of Honey Versus Sucrose on Appetite, Appetite-Regulating Hormones, and Postmeal Thermogenesis." *Journal of the American College of Nutrition* 29.5 (2010): 482–93.

5. Zamzil Amin Asha'ari et al. "Ingestion of Honey Improves the Symptoms of Allergic Rhinitis: Evidence from a Randomized Placebo-Controlled Trial in the East Coast of Peninsular Malaysia." *Annals of Saudi Medicine* 33.5 (2013): 469–75.

6. Manisha Deb Mandal and Shyamapada Mandal. "Honey: Its Medicinal Property and Antibacterial Activity." *Asian Pacific Journal of Tropical Biomedicine* 1.2 (2011): 154–60.

7. Rui Wang et al. "Honey's Ability to Counter Bacterial Infections Arises from Both Bactericidal Compounds and QS Inhibition." *Frontiers in Microbiology* 3 (2012): 144.

8. Sharon P. Fowler et al. "Fueling the Obesity Epidemic? Artificially Sweetened Beverage Use and Long-Term Weight Gain." *Obesity* 16.8 (2008): 1894–1900.

9. Sharon P. Fowler, Ken Williams, and Helen P. Hazuda. "Diet Soda Intake Is Associated with Long-Term Increases in Waist Circumference in a Biethnic Cohort of Older Adults: The San Antonio Longitudinal Study of Aging." *Journal of the American Geriatrics Society* 63.4 (2015): 708–15.

10. "Can an Ice Cream Diet Be Good for You?" ABC News; https://abcnews .go.com/GMA/story?id=125912&page=1. Accessed November 12, 2017.

CHAPTER 9. BE FREE OF FAT-FREE

1. Frank B. Hu, JoAnn E. Manson, and Walter C. Willett. "Types of Dietary Fat and Risk of Coronary Heart Disease: A Critical Review." *Journal of the American College of Nutrition* 20.1 (2001): 5–19.

2. Nicholas Bakalar. "New Study Favors Fat over Carbs." *New York Times*, September 8, 2017; https://www.nytimes.com/2017/09/08/well/new -study-favors-fat-over-carbs.html?mcubz=0. Accessed September 9, 2017.

3. Mahshid Dehghan et al. "Associations of Fats and Carbohydrate Intake with Cardiovascular Disease and Mortality in 18 Countries from Five Continents (PURE): A Prospective Cohort Study." *The Lancet* 390.10107 (2017): 2050–62.

4. "Fats and Cholesterol." The Nutrition Source, Harvard T. H. Chan School of Public Health; https://www.hsph.harvard.edu/nutritionsource/what -should-you-eat/fats-and-cholesterol/. Accessed April 30, 2017.

5. Christopher Ingraham. "The Average American Woman Now Weighs as Much as the Average 1960s Man." *Washington Post*, June 12, 2015; https://

www.washingtonpost.com/news/wonk/wp/2015/06/12/look-at-how
-much-weight-weve-gained-since-the-1960s/. Accessed September 9, 2017.

6. "Healthy Dietary Styles." The Nutrition Source, Harvard T. H. Chan School of Public Health; https://www.hsph.harvard.edu/nutritionsource /healthy-dietary-styles/. Accessed April 30, 2017.

7. Susanne Rautiainen et al. "Dairy Consumption in Association with Weight Change and Risk of Becoming Overweight or Obese in Middle-Aged and Older Women: A Prospective Cohort Study." *American Journal of Clinical Nutrition* 103.4 (2016): 979–88.

8. Mohammad Y. Yakoob et al. "Circulating Biomarkers of Dairy Fat and Risk of Incident Diabetes Mellitus Among U.S. Men and Women in Two Large Prospective Cohorts." *Circulation* 133.17 (2016): 1645–54.

9. Georg Loss et al. "The Protective Effect of Farm Milk Consumption on Childhood Asthma and Atopy: The GABRIELA Study." *Journal of Allergy and Clinical Immunology* 128.4 (2011): 766–73.

10. Mark Holbreich et al. "Amish Children Living in Northern Indiana Have a Very Low Prevalence of Allergic Sensitization." *Journal of Allergy and Clinical Immunology* 129.6 (2012): 1671–73.

11. Michael Pollan. *In Defense of Food.* New York: Penguin, 2010, Kindle Edition.

12. Cristin E. Kearns, Laura A. Schmidt, and Stanton A. Glantz. "Sugar Industry and Coronary Heart Disease Research: A Historical Analysis of Internal Industry Documents." *JAMA Internal Medicine* 176.11 (2016): 1680–85.

CHAPTER 10. BREAKING BREAD MYTHS

1. Benjamin Lebwohl et al. "Long-Term Gluten Consumption in Adults Without Celiac Disease and Risk of Coronary Heart Disease: Prospective Cohort Study." *BMJ* 357 (2017): j1892.

2. Dagfinn Aune et al. "Whole Grain Consumption and Risk of Cardiovascular Disease, Cancer, and All Cause and Cause Specific Mortality: Systematic Review and Dose-Response Meta-Analysis of Prospective Studies." *BMJ* 353 (2016): i2716.

Notes

3. Geng Zong et al. "Whole Grain Intake and Mortality from All Causes, Cardiovascular Disease, and Cancer: A Meta-Analysis of Prospective Cohort Studies." *Circulation* 133.24 (2016): 2370–80.

4. Joelle David. "Turns Out Eating Potatoes and Pasta Isn't Bad After All: Study." *New York Post*, May 9, 2018; https://nypost.com/2018/05/09/turns-out-eating -potatoes-and-pasta-isnt-bad-after-all-study/. Accessed June 4, 2018.

5. Ferris Jabr. "Bread Is Broken." *New York Times*, October 29, 2015; https: //www.nytimes.com/2015/11/01/magazine/bread-is-broken.html. Accessed July 22, 2017.

6. Jessica R. Biesiekierski et al. "Gluten Causes Gastrointestinal Symptoms in Subjects Without Celiac Disease: A Double-Blind Randomized Placebo-Controlled Trial." *American Journal of Gastroenterology* 106.3 (2011): 508–14.

7. Jessica R. Biesiekierski et al. "No Effects of Gluten in Patients with Self-Reported Non-Celiac Gluten Sensitivity After Dietary Reduction of Fermentable, Poorly Absorbed, Short-Chain Carbohydrates." *Gastroenterology* 145.2 (2013): 320–28.

8. Julia Moskin. "Rye, a Grain with Ancient Roots, Is Rising Again." *New York Times*, January 10, 2017; https://www.nytimes.com/2017/01/10/dining /rye-grain-bread.html. Accessed August 3, 2017.

CHAPTER 11. BREAK-FAST, DIET LESS

1. Hana Kahleova et al. "Meal Frequency and Timing Are Associated with Changes in Body Mass Index in Adventist Health Study 2." *Journal of Nutrition* 147.9 (2017): 1722–28.

2. Daniela Jakubowicz et al. "High Caloric Intake at Breakfast vs. Dinner Differentially Influences Weight Loss of Overweight and Obese Women." *Obesity* 21.12 (2013): 2504–12.

3. Roni Caryn Rabin. "The Case for a Breakfast Feast." *New York Times*, August 21, 2017; https://www.nytimes.com/2017/08/21/well/eat/the-case -for-a-breakfast-feast.html. Accessed October 10, 2017.

Notes

4. Megumi Hatori et al. "Time-Restricted Feeding Without Reducing Caloric Intake Prevents Metabolic Diseases in Mice Fed a High-Fat Diet." *Cell Metabolism* 15.6 (2012): 848–60.

5. "Skipping Breakfast Associated with Hardening of the Arteries." American College of Cardiology, October 2, 2017; http://www.acc.org/about-acc /press-releases/2017/10/02/13/56/skipping-breakfast-associated-with -hardening-of-the-arteries. Accessed June 3, 2018. Irina Uzhova et al. "The Importance of Breakfast in Atherosclerosis Disease: Insights from the PESA Study." *Journal of the American College of Cardiology* 70.15 (2017): 1833–42.

6. "Meal Planning, Timing, May Impact Heart Health." American Heart Association Scientific Statement, January 30, 2017; http://newsroom.heart .org/news/meal-planning-timing-may-impact-heart-health. Accessed October 10, 2017.

7. Alison Fildes et al. "Probability of an Obese Person Attaining Normal Body Weight: Cohort Study Using Electronic Health Records." *American Journal of Public Health* 105.9 (2015): e54–e59.

8. Shoaib Afzal et al. "Change in Body Mass Index Associated with Lowest Mortality in Denmark, 1976–2013." *JAMA* 315.18 (2016): 1989–96.

9. A. J. Tomiyama et al. "Misclassification of Cardiometabolic Health When Using Body Mass Index Categories in NHANES 2005–2012." *International Journal of Obesity* 40.5 (2016): 883–86.

10. David K. Li. "Crash Dieting Might Actually Make You Gain Weight." *New York Post*, April 10, 2018; https://nypost.com/2018/04/10/crash -dieting-might-actually-make-you-gain-weight/. Accessed June 4, 2018.

11. Dariush Mozaffarian et al. "Changes in Diet and Lifestyle and Long-Term Weight Gain in Women and Men." *New England Journal of Medicine* 364.25 (2011): 2392–404.

12. "The 90+ Study." UCI Mind; http://www.mind.uci.edu/research-studies /90plus-study/. Accessed June 4, 2018.

13. Ramón Estruch et al. "Primary Prevention of Cardiovascular Disease with a Mediterranean Diet." *New England Journal of Medicine* 368.14 (2013): 1279–90.

Notes

CHAPTER 12. SKIP TO THE GYM

1. Miranda E. G. Armstrong et al. "Frequent Physical Activity May Not Reduce Vascular Disease Risk as Much as Moderate Activity: Large Prospective Study of UK Women." *Circulation* 131.8 (2015): CirculationAHA.114.010296.

2. Charles E. Matthews et al. "Use of Time and Energy on Exercise, Prolonged TV Viewing, and Work Days." *American Journal of Preventive Medicine* 55.3 (2018): e61–e69.

3. Peter Schnohr et al. "Dose of Jogging and Long-Term Mortality: The Copenhagen City Heart Study." *Journal of the American College of Cardiology* 65.5 (2015): 411–19.

4. Alice Park. "When Exercise Does More Harm Than Good." *Time*, February 2, 2015; http://time.com/3692668/when-exercise-does-more-harm-than-good/. Accessed November 5, 2017.

5. Jenna B. Gillen et al. "Three Minutes of All-Out Intermittent Exercise per Week Increases Skeletal Muscle Oxidative Capacity and Improves Cardiometabolic Health." *PLOS One* 9.11 (2014): e111489.

6. Keith M. Diaz et al. "Patterns of Sedentary Behavior and Mortality in U.S. Middle-Aged and Older Adults: A National Cohort Study." *Annals of Internal Medicine* 167.7 (2017): 465–75.

7. "Science Agrees: Nature Is Good for You." Association of Nature and Forest Therapy Guides and Programs; http://www.natureandforesttherapy. org/the-science.html. Accessed November 5, 2017.

8. Bruce Neal. "Fat Chance for Physical Activity." *Population Health Metrics* 11.1 (2013): 9.

9. Aseem Malhotra. "Take Off That Fitbit: Exercise Alone Won't Make You Lose Weight." *Washington Post*, May 15, 2015; https://www.washington post.com/posteverything/wp/2015/05/15/take-off-that-fitbit-exercise -alone-wont-make-you-lose-weight/. Accessed November 5, 2017.

10. Joene Hendry. "Sitting Too Long May Be Dangerous for Young Infants." Reuters, May 13, 2008; https://www.reuters.com/article/us-sitting-infants

/sitting-too-long-may-be-dangerous-for-young-infants-idUSKEN
37119120080513. Accessed September 17, 2018.

CHAPTER 13. LET THE SUNSHINE IN

1. Robyn M. Lucas et al. "Estimating the Global Disease Burden Due to Ultraviolet Radiation Exposure." *International Journal of Epidemiology* 37.3 (2008): 654–67.

2. P. G. Lindqvist et al. "Avoidance of Sun Exposure as a Risk Factor for Major Causes of Death: A Competing Risk Analysis of the Melanoma in Southern Sweden Cohort." *Journal of Internal Medicine* 280.4 (2016): 375–87.

3. Centers for Disease Control and Prevention. "Skin Cancer—Sun Safety." https://www.cdc.gov/cancer/skin/basic_info/sun-safety.htm. Accessed July 3, 2017.

4. Rathish Nair and Arun Maseeh. "Vitamin D: The 'Sunshine' Vitamin." *Journal of Pharmacology & Pharmacotherapeutics* 3.2 (2012): 118–26.

5. Trude Eid Robsahm et al. "Vitamin D_3 from Sunlight May Improve the Prognosis of Breast, Colon and Prostate Cancer (Norway)." *Cancer Causes and Control* 15.2 (2004): 149–58.

6. Thieu X. Phan et al. "Intrinsic Photosensitivity Enhances Motility of T Lymphocytes." *Scientific Reports* 6 (2016): 39479.

7. Mohamed Boubekri et al. "Impact of Windows and Daylight Exposure on Overall Health and Sleep Quality of Office Workers: A Case-Control Pilot Study." *Journal of Clinical Sleep Medicine* 10.6 (2014): 603–11.

8. Jaymi Heimbuch. "How Watching Sunrise or Sunset Can Improve Your Health." MNN.com19, November 19, 2015; https://www.mnn.com/health/fitness-well-being/blogs/how-watching-sunrise-or-sunset-can-improve-your-health. Accessed June 4, 2018.

Notes

CHAPTER 14. EAT OLD (FERMENTED) FOOD

1. Maria L. Marco et al. "Health Benefits of Fermented Foods: Microbiota and Beyond." *Current Opinion in Biotechnology* 44 (2017): 94–102.

2. Eva M. Selhub, Alan C. Logan, and Alison C. Bested. "Fermented Foods, Microbiota, and Mental Health: Ancient Practice Meets Nutritional Psychiatry." *Journal of Physiological Anthropology* 33.1 (2014): 2.

3. Felice N. Jacka et al. "Association of Western and Traditional Diets with Depression and Anxiety in Women." *American Journal of Psychiatry* 167.3 (2010): 305–11.

4. Almundena Sánchez-Villegas et al. "Association of the Mediterranean Dietary Pattern with the Incidence of Depression: The Seguimiento Universidad de Navarra/University of Navarra Follow-up (SUN) Cohort." *Archives of General Psychiatry* 66.10 (2009): 1090–98.

CHAPTER 15. BREASTFEEDING IS BEST FEEDING

1. Jill Krasny. "Nestle's Infant Formula Scandal." *Business Insider*, June 25, 2012; http://www.businessinsider.com/nestles-infant-formula-scandal -2012-6. Accessed October 12, 2017.

2. Edward Baer. "Babies Means Business." *New Internationalist*, April 1, 1982; https://newint.org/features/1982/04/01/babies. Accessed October 12, 2017.

3. Centers for Disease Control and Prevention. "Breastfeeding: Frequently Asked Questions (FAQs)." June 16, 2015; https://www.cdc.gov/breastfeeding/faq/. Accessed September 26, 2017.

4. Mandy Oaklander. "Breastfeeding Linked to a Lower Risk of Cancer in Kids." *Time*, June 1, 2015; http://time.com/3901565/breastfeeding -childhood-cancer-leukemia/. Accessed October 7, 2017.

5. Joanna S. Hawkes, Mark A. Neumann, and Robert A. Gibson. "The Effect of Breast Feeding on Lymphocyte Subpopulations in Healthy Term Infants at 6 Months of Age." *Pediatric Research* 45.5 Pt 1 (1999): 648–51.

Notes

6. Jack Gilbert and Rob Knight. *Dirt Is Good: The Advantage of Germs for Your Child's Developing Immune System.* New York: St. Martin's Press, 2017, Kindle Edition.

7. American Institute for Cancer Research. "Diet, Nutrition, Physical Activity and Breast Cancer 2017." Revised 2018; http://www.aicr.org /continuous-update-project/reports/breast-cancer-report-2017.pdf? _ga=2.161086461.1517247984.1538262749-112444945.1538262748. Accessed October 3, 2018.

8. Susannah Brown. "Can Breastfeeding Help Prevent Breast Cancer?" World Cancer Research Fund International, July 31, 2017; http://www .wcrf.org/int/blog/articles/2017/07/can-breastfeeding-help-prevent-breast -cancer. Accessed October 3, 2017.

9. Efrat L. Amitay and Lital Keinan-Boker. "Breastfeeding and Childhood Leukemia Incidence: A Meta-Analysis and Systematic Review." *JAMA Pediatrics* 169.6 (2015): e151025.

10. Brown, "Can Breastfeeding Help Prevent Breast Cancer?"

11. Centers for Disease Control and Prevention. "Breast-Feeding Rates Continue to Rise." CDC Online Newsroom, August 22, 2016; https://www .cdc.gov/media/releases/2016/p0822-breast-feeding-rates.html. Accessed September 26, 2017.

12. World Health Organization. "Breastfeeding." http://www.who.int/nutrition /topics/exclusive_breast-feeding/en/. Accessed October 7, 2017.

13. L. Bricker, N. Medley, and J. J. Pratt. "Routine Ultrasound in Late Pregnancy (After 24 Weeks' Gestation)." *Cochrane Database of Systematic Reviews* 6 (2015): Art. No. CD001451. DOI: 10.1002/14651858.CD001451.pub4. J. Tieu et al. "Screening for Gestational Diabetes Mellitus Based on Different Risk Profiles and Settings for Improving Maternal and Infant Health." *Cochrane Database of Systematic Reviews* 8 (2017): Art. No. CD007222. DOI: 10.1002/14651858.CD007222.pub4.

CHAPTER 16. GET DOWN AND DIRTY

1. Michelle M. Stein et al. "Innate Immunity and Asthma Risk in Amish and Hutterite Farm Children." *New England Journal of Medicine* 375.5 (2016): 411–21.

2. Markus J. Ege et al. "Exposure to Environmental Microorganisms and Childhood Asthma." *New England Journal of Medicine* 364.8 (2011): 701–709.

3. Stephanie J. Lynch, Malcolm R. Sears, and Robert J. Hancox. "Thumb-Sucking, Nail-Biting, and Atopic Sensitization, Asthma, and Hay Fever." *Pediatrics* (2016): e20160443.

4. Matthew T. Walker et al. "Mechanism for Initiation of Food Allergy: Dependence on Skin Barrier Mutations and Environmental Allergen Costimulation." *Journal of Allergy and Clinical Immunology* 141.5 (2018): 1711–25.

5. Albert Barberán et al. "The Ecology of Microscopic Life in Household Dust." *Proceedings of the Royal Society B*: Biological Sciences 282.1814 (2015).

6. Jack Gilbert and Rob Knight. *Dirt Is Good: The Advantage of Germs for Your Child's Developing Immune System*. New York: St. Martin's Press, 2017, Kindle Edition.

7. Bill Hesselmar, Anna Hicke-Roberts, and Göran Wennergren. "Allergy in Children in Hand Versus Machine Dishwashing." *Pediatrics* 135.3 (2015): e590–e597.

8. Justin Sonnenburg and Erica Sonnenburg. *The Good Gut: Taking Control of Your Weight, Your Mood, and Your Long-Term Health*. New York: Penguin, 2015, Kindle Edition.

9. "ACI Statement on FDA Consumer Rule on Antibacterial Soaps." American Cleaning Institute, September 2, 2016; http://www.cleaninginstitute .org/aci_statement_on_fda_consumer_rule_on_antibacterial_soaps/. Accessed October 14, 2017.

10. Helena Helmby. "Human Helminth Therapy to Treat Inflammatory Disorders—Where Do We Stand?" *BMC Immunology* 16.1 (2015): 12.

11. "Fecal Transplantation (Bacteriotherapy)." Johns Hopkins Medicine, Gastroenterology and Hepatology; http://www.hopkinsmedicine.org/gastro enterology_hepatology/clinical_services/advanced_endoscopy/fecal _transplantation.html. Accessed October 21, 2017.

CHAPTER 17. HAPPINESS: PURSUE IT

1. Norman Cousins. *Anatomy of an Illness as Perceived by the Patient: Reflections on Healing and Regeneration*. New York: Open Road Media, 2016, Kindle Edition.

2. Alia J. Crum and Ellen J. Langer. "Mind-Set Matters: Exercise and the Placebo Effect." *Psychological Science* 18.2 (2007): 165–71.

3. Laura M. Hsu, Jaewoo Chung, and Ellen J. Langer. "The Influence of Age-Related Cues on Health and Longevity." *Perspectives on Psychological Science* 5.6 (2010): 632–48.

4. Bruce Grierson. "What if Age Is Nothing but a Mind-Set?" *New York Times*, October 22, 2014; https://www.nytimes.com/2014/10/26/magazine /what-if-age-is-nothing-but-a-mind-set.html. Accessed October 24, 2017.

5. "Is Broken Heart Syndrome Real?" American Heart Association, April 18, 2016; http://www.heart.org/en/health-topics/cardiomyopathy/what-is -cardiomyopathy-in-adults/is-broken-heart-syndrome-real. Accessed October 22, 2017.

6. "So Lonely I Could Die." American Psychological Association, August 5, 2017; http://www.apa.org/news/press/releases/2017/08/lonely-die.aspx. Accessed September 16, 2017.

7. Joshua Wolf Shenk. "What Makes Us Happy?" *The Atlantic*, June 2009; https://www.theatlantic.com/magazine/archive/2009/06/what-makes-us -happy/307439/. Accessed October 22, 2017.

8. Stacey Colino. "The Health Benefits of Hugging." *U.S. News & World Report*, February 3, 2016; https://health.usnews.com/health-news/health -wellness/articles/2016-02-03/the-health-benefits-of-hugging. Accessed October 30, 2017.

9. Adam Piore. "What Technology Can't Change About Happiness." *Nautilus,* September 17, 2015; http://nautil.us/issue/28/2050/what-technology -cant-change-about-happiness. Accessed October 22, 2017.

10. Michael Winnick. "Putting a Finger on Our Phone Obsession" dscout, June 16, 2016; https://blog.dscout.com/mobile-touches. Accessed October 22, 2017.

11. "Health Experts Recommend Standing Up at Desk, Leaving Office, Never Coming Back." *The Onion,* February 6, 2015; https://www.theonion.com /health-experts-recommend-standing-up-at-desk-leaving-o-1819577456. Accessed June 4, 2018.

12. Ben Steverman. "Retirement in America: We're Working Longer, Getting Sicker, and Dying Sooner." *Boston Globe,* October 23, 2017; https://www .bostonglobe.com/business/2017/10/23/retirement-america-working -longer-getting-sicker-and-dying-sooner/Onmy9PBfWx0x3WP4fjsTKP /story.html. Accessed October 24, 2017.

13. Bette Liu et al. "Does Happiness Itself Directly Affect Mortality? The Prospective U.K. Million Women Study." *The Lancet* 387.10021 (2016): 874–81.

14. Raeleen D'Agostino Mautner. *Living La Dolce Vita: Bring the Passion, Laughter, and Serenity of Italy into Your Daily Life.* Napierville, IL: Sourcebooks, 2003, p. xxiii.

AFTERWORD

1. "World's Oldest Man Israel Kristal, a Holocaust Survivor, Dies at 113 in Israel." New York *Daily News,* August 11, 2017; http://www.nydailynews .com/news/world/world-oldest-man-yisrael-kristal-dies-113-article -1.3403895. Accessed October 29, 2017.

ABOUT THE AUTHORS

DR. HARRY OFGANG is a native of Brooklyn who began his study of medicine at the Università di Perugia Medicina e Chirurgia (University of Perugia Faculty of Medicine and Surgery) before graduating from the National University of Natural Medicine in Portland, Oregon. In his thirty-eight-plus years practicing natural medicine, he has studied and lectured with some of natural medicine's most renowned figures, including friends and mentors Professor Francisco Eizayaga and George Vithoulkas. In the 1980s, he founded Hahnemann Health Associates on Park Avenue in New York City and Hahnemann Natural Health and Education Associates in Connecticut, both pioneering natural health and education centers. He is a sought-after lecturer and practitioner of homeopathic and naturopathic medicine.

ERIK OFGANG is a senior writer at *Connecticut Magazine*, where he writes frequently about health, science, food, and beer. He is the author of *Buzzed: Beers, Booze, and Coffee Brews* and *Gillette Castle: A History*. He has written for the Associated Press, *Tablet Magazine*, and

Thrillist, and he has taught journalism at Quinnipiac University, Mercy College, and at Western Connecticut State University's MFA in Creative and Professional Writing program. When he's not writing or teaching writing, he can be seen playing bass with the Celtic rock band MacTalla Mor.